Shape Up!

Shape Up!

An Aerobic-based
Home Work-out Programme

Maureen Hudson with Tom Mercer

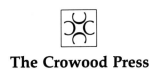

The Crowood Press

First published in 1989 by
The Crowood Press
Ramsbury, Marlborough,
Wiltshire SN8 2HE

British Library Cataloguing in Publication Data

Hudson, Maureen
 Shape Up! An Aerobic-based Home Work-out Programme
 1. Physical fitness. Aerobics
 I. Title   II. Mercer, Tom
 612.7'1

 ISBN 1 85223 189 0

Typeset by Avonset, Midsomer Norton, Bath.
Printed in Great Britain by The Bath Press.

Contents

Acknowledgements

I would like to thank the following friends and business associates for their support, influence and help whilst writing this book: my friend Sue Harding, for tirelessly typing away for hours – both speedily and professionally; my family, for their considerable and invaluable support, for their enthusiasm, their sharing and caring about my work, helping me to get through it all under great pressure and helping me make this book become a reality – with their support it gave me a feeling of pride in introducing you to the exciting field of physical fitness.

Introduction

In developed countries the late twentieth century has seen the manifestation of two definite trends in society. One of these is the clearly reduced amount of regular physical activity in the community at large. 'Hi-tech' developments in industry and the changing nature of employment (the growth of service industries and the decline of traditional manufacturing industries) have accelerated the 'redundancy' of high levels of occupational physical activity. In addition to such declining emphasis upon physical activity at work, it is also recognised that 'sedentarism' pervades much of our non-working time. As a nation we tend to be transported to and from work (by car or public transport), we tend to choose the lifts or escalator in preference to the stairs and when we relax we tend to slump in front of the television, becoming a society of 'passive' consumers of leisure.

In conjunction with this trend of increased physical inactivity it is now widely recognised that lifestyle-related problems are the new threat to public health. Where once the fear of infectious diseases (related to poor public hygiene and housing) loomed large, this has now been replaced by public health problems (including coronary heart disease, high blood pressure, obesity, certain forms of diabetes, low back pain, and osteoporosis), some of whose origins can be traced to a variety of 'cultural pollutants' which are prevalent in developed countries. Such pollutants include substance-abuse (tobacco, alcohol and drugs), inadequate and/or inappropriate nutrition and importantly *physical inactivity*! In fact, some health statistics attribute the cause of over fifty per cent of all premature deaths to lifestyle-related factors!

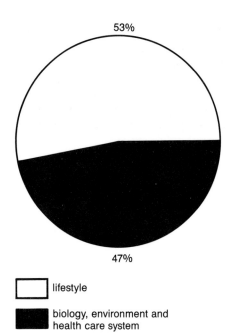

53%

47%

lifestyle

biology, environment and health care system

Factors implicated as causes of premature death.

Many of these lifestyle-related health problems (such as those listed above) have been termed *hypokinetic* diseases or disorders in recognition of the fact that physical inactivity has been fairly firmly linked with either the onset or aggravation of the conditions. As a consequence of the temporal coincidence of these two trends and the reported links between them, many people are beginning to examine the possibility of incorporating physical activity into *their* lives. Of necessity this involves reorganisation of their leisure or non-working time. For some of us this will not be a problem since we may already be convinced of the benefits of exercise. Equally importantly we may have easy access to good facilities and in addition we may already be fairly well informed about exercise. However, for many others the adjustment of their daily routine to accommodate a regular exercise session appears to pose both real and imaginary problems. The contrasting responses to the idea of incorporating exercise into our daily routines can perhaps be illustrated by reference to the table below which examines some of the reasons why some people do and some people do not take up exercise.

Justification given for, and excuses made for not, exercising

Justifications
health and fitness (No. 1)
enjoyment
physical appearance (women in particular)
as a means of relaxation and stress release
Excuses
don't have the time/too inconvenient
lack of facilities
bad weather

Because some of the most commonly cited reasons for not exercising are unlikely to change overnight (if access to facilities is a problem today, it is likely to be a problem tomorrow), and because they are indeed important stumbling-blocks to the adoption of, and adherence to, regular exercise, we have decided to construct a *home-based* exercise programme around the popular and flexible exercise activity of aerobics. In essence what we are presenting is a comprehensive package of material which will provide:

1. some of the reasons why you should exercise (the health benefits of exercise);
2. guidelines for conditioning (or how to get the best out of yourself and your exercise programme);
3. detailed instruction in all aspects of the aerobics exercise workout (including an extensive range of exercise activities).

WHY EXERCISE?

The number one reason given for exercising (or even 'threatening' to exercise) is that people believe it will improve their health and/or physical fitness. Both these concepts (health and physical fitness) are ones most people use and refer to in everyday life – but what exactly do we mean when we use them, and more importantly, what is the real meaning of each of the terms?

Quite often we describe people as being healthy and/or fit and we may even use both terms interchangeably. The obvious interpretation of such behaviour is that for many people the concepts may be considered as being the same thing, or at least interrelated. In actual fact however health tends to be defined as a concept 'encompassing physical and mental fitness, and general well-being, as well as freedom from disease (it is therefore multidimensional in nature reflecting social, mental, emotional, spiritual, and physical facets)'.

Fitness on the other hand is a concept which has many interpretations but is usually thought of as a word describing 'one's capabilities to participate effectively in specific tasks (for example fit to work, fit to run for the bus and so forth)'. Recently, however, physical fitness has been defined as 'a set of attributes that people have or achieve that relates to the ability to perform physical activity'.

As you can see, there are indeed areas of overlap between these definitions, but equally obviously you can see definite distinctions (and thus differences) between them. You may be wondering what all this means?

Essentially it means that people should be aware that physical fitness and improved health are interrelated but not synonymous. Whilst it is probably true to say that in order to achieve very high levels of physical fitness you usually require good health, it is not, however, the case that improvements in physical fitness will insure increased health or immunity to disease. However evidence is accumulating fairly rapidly that the incorporation of appropriate exercise into your lifestyle can help you achieve the state of 'wellness' – a concept developed in America which describes 'a state of well-being where people are operating at or near their potential because of the lifestyle they have adopted. (It is also described as the integration of components of health, and is therefore much more than just the avoidance of illness).'

The adoption of regular and appropriate exercise habits and/or the improvement of physical fitness, as a means of developing wellness, have both been implicated in the achievement of the health benefits of exercise. However, before examining these benefits it is appropriate to clarify further what is (and indeed can be) meant by physical fitness. As outlined above this concept involves the 'possession' of certain attributes (characteristics) that relate to the ability of individuals to perform physical activity. These attributes have been described as being 'given' or 'achievable' and refer to aspects of our physiology and physical performance capacity which are determined by inherited characteristics and/or our exercise endeavours (conditioning). Furthermore, physical fitness can be sub-divided into skill-related fitness and health-related sub-components (see the table below which lists the components of physical fitness).

Health-related components
1. cardiorespiratory endurance
2. muscular strength
3. muscular endurance
4. flexibility
5. body composition
6. stress management

Skill-related components
1. agility
2. speed
3. power
4. co-ordination
5. balance
6. reaction time

With regard to the 'given' or 'achieved' contribution to your physical fitness it is generally recognised that the skill-related components are, to a great extent, genetically determined. Furthermore, while they are undoubtedly important components of fitness, their use is mainly evident in the sport performance arena – there is no evidence linking any of these aspects of fitness with health or wellness. Improvements in the health-related components of fitness, however, have been linked with enhanced wellness.

THE COMPONENTS OF HEALTH-RELATED FITNESS (HRF)

Cardiorespiratory Endurance

This component of HRF reflects the condition (health and fitness) of the heart, associated blood vessels and lungs to provide adequate transport of oxygen to the exercising muscles in order that the muscles can 'burn' their fuel to produce energy for exercise.

Cardiorespiratory fitness can only be developed if individuals engage in exercise which involves the large muscle groups of the body (such as the legs) in rhythmic and dynamic movement. This type of movement pattern will cause individuals to increase their rate of energy expenditure, but will also ensure that the energy requirements of the exercise are met aerobically. This means that the fuels for energy release during exercise will be 'burned' in the presence of oxygen. Aerobic energy release is considered to be both more efficient and desirable than anaerobic energy release (which does not involve oxygen).

This can be explained by the fact that individuals can only call on anaerobic energy-release processes for a few minutes at the most, whereas they can sustain aerobic energy production for hours. Consequently we would expect indivduals with high levels of cardiorespiratory endurance to be those people with an enhanced capacity to 'burn' fuel aerobically – thus possessing a high aerobic capacity (a measure of cardiorespiratory endurance and a reflection, in part, of the adoption of regular aerobic exercise). This enhanced capacity is reflected in the ability of individuals to participate for longer periods in such activities and so provides them with the potential to lead more active lives.

The specific benefits of regular participation in exercise likely to improve cardiorespiratory endurance include:

1. a strengthened heart muscle which increases the efficiency of the heart as a pump;
2. an increase in the number of blood vessels supplying the heart and muscles;
3. a reduction in the resistance to flow (blood pressure);
4. an increase in the total volume of blood and its capacity to carry oxygen;
5. an improved lung efficiency;
6. improved energy production within the muscle;
7. improved oxygen extraction by the muscle.

There are also other associated benefits, including:

1. a reduced risk of some aspects of heart disease;

2. an enhanced ability to withstand emotional stress;
3. enhanced 'weight control' (body fat management – *see* body composition).

Muscular Strength and Endurance

The development and maintenance of muscular strength (MS) and endurance (ME) is an integral part of a comprehensive HRF programme. MS refers to the ability of the body (or any of its parts, such as muscles) to apply force against a heavy resistance (weight). ME, on the other hand, is the ability to repeatedly carry out muscular tasks over a period of time.

Any exercise programme which incorporates these components of HRF would be helping to combat the loss of lean tissue (muscle mass) associated with inactivity. It has been reported that as this loss of muscle tissue occurs, individuals may in fact be predisposed to chronic low back pain. Furthermore, such loss of lean tissue has also been associated with a reduction in metabolic rate, which can lead to increased fat deposition. As an additional consequence of muscular inactivity researchers have indicated that bones may lose strength. This decrease in bone strength has been associated with the development of osteoporosis and all that this may entail (possible hip and vertebral fractures). This condition is particularly prevalent in the post-menopausal female. It is interesting to note that evidence is beginning to accumulate to support the view that weight-bearing exercise of a muscular-endurance type is beneficial in reducing the likelihood of this condition.

Flexibility

Flexibility is the term we use to refer to the range of movement (ROM) about a joint. This

ROM is greatly determined – and so limited – by the structures surrounding and indeed composing our joints (muscles, tendons, ligaments and skin). Inactivity and ageing are both associated with a decrease in flexibility. This is thought to occur as a result of muscles and tendons becoming less supple. However, because the soft tissues which support and surround the joints are elastic, exercise can partially restore this suppleness. Stretching exercises are particularly useful for this purpose. However, unless these exercises are performed regularly these soft tissues (muscles in particular) will lose their suppleness and return to being stiff and tight.

There are a number of stretching techniques available, but it is generally recognised that static stretches should be employed as these are known to cause fewer injuries. This involves stretching the muscle slowly and gradually until the point of mild discomfort and then holding that position for 15–30 seconds. This is a controlled and safe form of stretching. Flexibility is joint-specific – meaning that each joint will have a unique potential ROM due to the configuration of tissues around it and the amount and type of use it gets. Consequently a good stretching programme should attempt to regularly work each joint through its full ROM.

This component of HRF is also an important part of the total work-out for all-round health/fitness. Appropriately chosen and properly executed, stretching exercises are considered able to improve muscle tone and prevent injuries. Additionally they are reported to improve body performance by enhancing circulation, body mobility, flexibility and in some cases strength. It has also been claimed that such exercises promote more restful sleep, more effective digestion of food, less depression or nervous tension and less muscle and joint pain (particularly low back pain).

Body Composition (weight control)

Body composition, or more accurately body leanness, is a very important part of HRF. This area of HRF is not without some confusion, especially with regard to exactly what is meant by 'weight control'. The use of the term overweight to describe someone who is carrying more than a few kilograms of excess fat is misleading. This term was coined to describe those individuals who were observed to possess a 'heavier than average body-weight for their height' (according to standard height–weight charts). Most of us will have used such tables at some time in order to find out if our current weight is desirable for our stature. Some insurance companies still use such methods to assess risk of premature death as a result of obesity. However, it is the condition of overfatness (obesity) with which we should be concerned. Furthermore, since such tables only look at the 'whole package' they tell us nothing about our current levels of body fat. The list, below, summarises some of the important terms associated with this component of HRF.

Body composition The combination of bone, fat and muscle tissue.
Body fat 'Essential' fat required for living and non-essential storage fat.
Lean body mass (fat free weight) The weight of fat-free tissue: muscle, bone, organs and skin.
Overweight Total body-weight in excess of an established height–weight standard.
Obesity The excessive accumulation of body fat, regardless of weight.

Being overfat poses more severe problems than merely having clothes which do not fit. Obesity has been linked with a number of diseases including coronary heart disease, hypertension (high blood pressure) and dia-

11

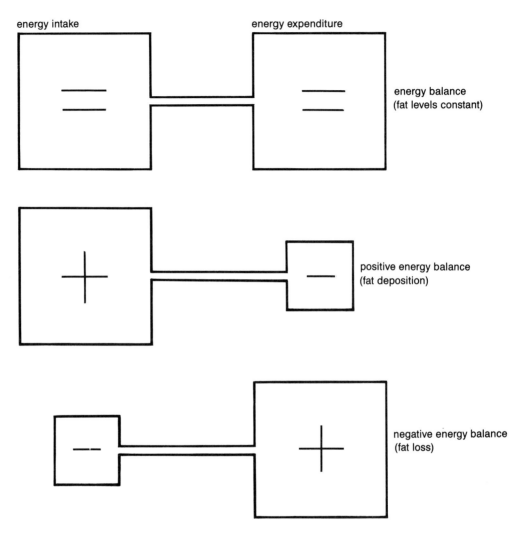

Energy balance and imbalance (after Brooks and Fahey, 1985).

betes. You may be asking yourself one of the following questions at this point: how do I avoid becoming overfat? – or; as I am presently overfat, how do I get rid of it? – or; how much fat should I ideally have? The answer to the first two questions can be explained by referring to the diagram above. This illustrates that weight – or more accurately fat – control is governed by a simple equation involving energy intake (food and drink consumed) and energy expenditure (the level of physical activity). It is interesting to note that overfatness tends to be the result of physical inactivity (low energy expenditure) rather than excessive eating (high energy intake)!

It is generally agreed that a combination of aerobic exercise and prudent eating habits will ensure weight (fat) control. Furthermore,

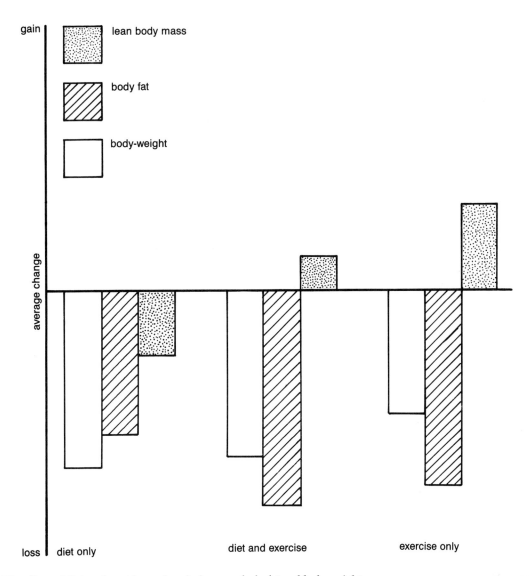

The effects of diet and exercise on lean body mass, body fat and body-weight.

fat loss is best achieved through a combination of increased aerobic exercise and modest dietary restriction (this is illustrated above). This type of exercise will aid fat control by:

1. increasing the overall level of energy expenditure;

2. increasing the proportion of fat used during exercise;

3. elevating the basal metabolic rate for several hours after exercise;

4. specifically reducing the total amount of body fat.

An important point to take in here is that it is actually more desirable to work at relatively low intensities of exercise (*see* the guidelines for conditioning) for prolonged periods of time if fat reduction is your aim. This is to be recommended as high-intensity exercise demands that the body switch over its fuel supply from fats to carbohydrates. Therefore your aim should be generally to increase the amount of time that you spend in moderate aerobic activity. Yet another key point to understand is that as we get older, we need to eat less because our basal metabolic rate slows down. However, what invariably happens as we age is that we continue to eat the same amounts (energy intake remains constant), exercise less (energy expenditure declines), and in addition to this we are faced with a slowing basal metabolic rate (meaning we need even less energy for 'resting body functions'). As a consequence we gradually accumulate a positive energy balance – with the result that we become fat!

It is therefore important to appreciate that this 'creeping obesity' – and that is exactly what it is – can be controlled by modest reductions in energy intake and adherence to regular aerobic exercise as we age. With regard to optimal levels of body fat, the following presents a summary of current thinking.

	Percentage body fat	
	MEN	WOMEN
Most athletes	5–13	12–22
Optimal health	10–20	18–25
Optimal fitness	10–18	16–25
Obesity	>25	>30

THE HEALTH BENEFITS OF EXERCISE

As explained above the achievement of the state of physical fitness involves a complex interaction between our inherited characteristics and our exercise habits. It is important to realise, however, that the health benefits associated with exercise are derived from the 'doing' and not necessarily the 'being'. In

fitness component	proposed health benefit	evidence
muscular strength/endurance	improved posture	+ +
	reduced low back pain	+
	decreased osteoporosis	+
flexibility	improved posture	+
	reduced low back pain	+
	decreased injury chance	+
aerobic exercise	reduced risk of heart disease	+ +
	reduced obesity	+ +
	decreased high blood pressure (in moderate hypertensives)	+
	reduced depression/anxiety	+
	controlled type II diabetes	+

The proposed health benefits of health-related fitness (and associated activity).

simple terms the key message is that it is the adoption and maintenance of regular and appropriate exercise habits which brings about any likely health benefits. Whilst a high level of physical fitness (assessed by a fitness-test score, perhaps) is a desirable feature, it is important to appreciate that this will reflect the combined contributions of our inherited characteristics (over which we have no control) and our exercise habits. As a result some people may be assessed as being very fit on the basis of a physical fitness-test score, which may actually be reflecting a combination of fortunate genetic endowment and poor exercise habits. Alternatively, individuals with moderate genetic endowment and good exercise habits may only score moderately on a test of physical fitness. Furthermore, it is well documented that fitness is a transitory phenomenon – which means if you don't use it, you really will lose it! Therefore on the basis of physical fitness classification (test score) alone, you cannot adequately measure health status. However, what can be said with some degree of certainty is that regular participation in exercise sessions which incorporate elements of all the components of HRF will enhance the achievement of wellness. Modifying a well-worn but nonetheless apposite maxim the evidence seems to suggest that 'regular exercise will add life to our years, and may indeed add years to our lives'.

GUIDELINES FOR CONDITIONING

Having examined some of the reasons which might explain why we should be thinking of developing our health-related fitness, we now need to turn our attention towards the general and specific guidelines which may help us to achieve this.

General Guidelines

The general guidelines are more commonly known as the principles of exercise conditioning. Basically there are three principles or guidelines which need to be considered in the design of your home-based work-out programme and these are:

1. overload;
2. progression;
3. specificity.

All types of exercise conditioning are governed by these principles, and it is the application of these which forms the physiological basis for the development of your own exercise conditioning programme. Scientific evidence has demonstrated time and again that consistent conditioning which takes into account individual differences (age, initial fitness and so forth) and adheres to these fundamental principles will promote optimal gains in exercise performance capacity (fitness) – according to each individual's genetic potential.

Overload

The principle of overload is the cornerstone of exercise conditioning and is acknowledged as being the key to the achievement of virtually all physical fitness and health benefits. Incorporating overload into any programme means that exercise carried out must be stressful enough (in a positive manner) to stimulate the desired physiological and physical changes in the body. The extent of the overloading does not need to be great, but it should repeatedly place an increasing demand upon the tissues/organs of the body. The essence of this principle is to do a little more in your exercise session today than you did in the last one, and in the next one aim to do just a little more again.

15

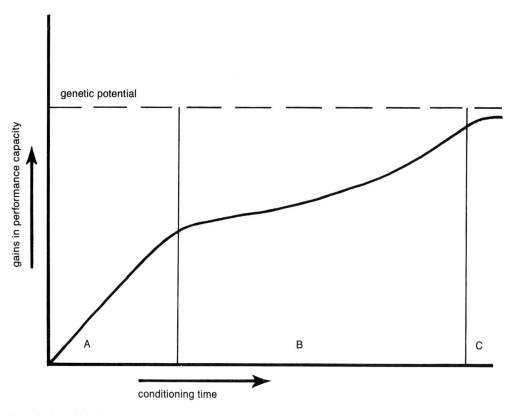

The theoretical conditioning curve.

It is important to appreciate that the effects of overload (and conditioning in general) will not be the same for all people. Furthermore, the way in which our body will adapt to these new demands placed upon it will be determined by the following factors:

1. the type of exercise we engage in;
2. the amount of exercise we do (amount = frequency × duration);
3. the intensity at which we choose to exercise.

Although individual differences will be apparent in our response to the stimulus of exercise, it is also true to say that most people will experience three distinct phases in their adaptation to this stimulus. These phases are perhaps best illustrated by reference to the above illustration which depicts a theoretical conditioning curve.

Generally, as individuals begin to exercise (especially if they have not had a history of previous activity) they can expect initial gains in exercise performance capacity to be relatively large and quite quickly achieved. Phase A of the graph illustrates that time and effort invested in conditioning are almost linearly reflected in improvements. As the curve enters phase B we can see that both the rate and size of improvement is beginning to decrease. This indicates that further progress can only be made at a much slower rate and with relatively more effort being required to achieve relatively smaller increments of improvement in exercise performance capacity. Eventually, as we enter phase C, we are approaching our genetic ceiling in terms of exercise performance capacity; the graph is now depicting the stage of diminishing returns, where even fairly modest improvements can only be achieved (if at all) as a result of a wholly disproportionate investment in terms of both time and effort. Essentially the basic shape of this conditioning curve will be the same for most people – but the ceiling (imposed by genetic potential) and thus the magnitude of potential gains – will vary considerably.

It is generally accepted that overload should be created initially in terms of the amount of exercise undertaken. This can be achieved by increasing the number of exercise sessions per week (frequency) and/or the length of time you spend exercising in each session (duration). It is only when you feel comfortable working out more frequently and for longer periods of time that you should consider increasing the intensity of the work-out. More specific information will be presented in the specific guidelines section, on the following page, but if we take aerobic exercise, the core element in the work-out, as an example see the recommended guidelines for conditioning below.

Basically we do not advise increasing the exercise intensity until you can comfortably complete at least three exercise sessions per week, incorporating aerobic components of 30–40 minutes' duration. It should also be

appreciated that conditioning gains can and will be lost just as rapidly as they were acquired if you stop exercising. This is known as the principle of reversibility; basically this reminds us that we cannot 'store' fitness.

Progression

The application of this principle demands that individuals become aware that the readjustment of overload, which needs to be made, must be applied in a manner which will allow the body to adjust and adapt to the new stimulus. Consequently, if gradual progressive overloading is accomplished, the body will adapt positively. However, if the overload is too great in extent and/or too rapid in rate, there is a strong likelihood that fatigue, muscle soreness and possible injury may occur.

This is not a rare occurrence as most people are tempted to adopt this 'too much too soon' approach in their impatience to progress. The guiding principle here should be 'listen to your body'. If you feel unduly tired or sore after an exercise session than you have probably done too much, so take it easier in your next session and make sure you have a day off in between sessions.

Specificity

This principle can be summed up by the statement; 'you will gain what you train'. In simple terms this refers to the fact that conditioning adaptations are specific to:

	Beginner	Advanced
Frequency:	3 × week	5 × week
Duration	20 mins per session	30–60 mins per session
Intensity	60–75% Max Heart Rate Reserve (MHRR)	75–90% MHRR

Recommended guidelines for conditioning.

1. the body parts being conditioned;
2. the component of health-related fitness being stressed.

Consequently, aerobic conditioning will not lead to improvement in flexibility. Similarly, improving the exercise performance capacity of the legs will not lead to increased capacity of the arms.

SPECIFIC GUIDELINES FOR CONDITIONING

Warm-up

Each of your work-out sessions should begin with a warm-up period of some 10–15 minutes to prepare the body for the more vigorous, aerobic component of the exercise session. The term warm-up is commonly used to describe those activities (generally consisting of light aerobic exercise, static stretching and some mobility exercises) which specifically prepare the heart, lungs and muscles for such exertion. This is achieved by performing low-intensity 'limbering-up' exercises which if carried out properly will:

1. increase both body temperature and the temperature of the muscles;
2. increase the transport of blood to the working muscles, thus enhancing oxygen delivery and allowing full aerobic energy production to take place;
3. increase the heart rate, thus preparing the cardiovascular system for work;
4. prepare the muscles and joints for more demanding activity;
5. set you up mentally for the core component of your work-out.

It is important to get the intensity and duration of the warm-up just right for you. An insufficient warm-up accomplishes nothing, whilst overdoing it may lead to fatigue before you can complete the total work-out. The onset of light sweating is a good indication that you are working at the correct level. To help in this process it is advisable to wear additional clothing for the warm-up. The extra layer(s) of clothing will prevent some of the heat loss from your body until your muscles are adequately warmed up. As the warm-up proceeds you will want to remove these additional items of clothing, so loose-fitting garments are best. A tracksuit is ideal but an old sweater can perform the same function.

It is recommended that the cardiovascular (temperature raising) portion of the warm-up should always precede the static stretching component. This is due to the fact that the muscles will be more receptive to stretching when their temperature has been raised.

Cool-down

Just as it is important to have a gradual and controlled transition from rest to exercise (warm-up), so it is equally important to ensure that the transition from exercise back to the resting state is similarly controlled and gradual (cool-down). Unfortunately, although the benefits and indeed importance of the cool-down have been well documented in academic literature, this component of the total work-out is often ignored by exercisers. Do not let this be the case with you!

After exercising many people stop immediately and either sit down or head for the showers. In these instances of exercise ending abruptly, the blood which has been redirected to the working muscles during exercise often 'pools' there, with the result that less blood is returned to the heart. This can cause dizziness and fainting and may in some instances 'shock' the heart. Think of the guardsman who may faint after being on parade for a long time; he has been standing in the same position for quite a while and as a result the blood collects in his legs. Because of this insufficient amounts of blood return to the heart with every beat and so the brain itself receives an inadequate supply. However, if the same guardsman were to march up and down for a few paces every now and then, the muscular activity in the legs would drive sufficient blood back to the heart. To counteract the pooling of blood which can accompany the abrupt termination of exercise, it is recommended that the aerobic component of the work-out is followed by 5–6 minutes lighter activity (walking round the room will suffice). The key point is that this activity provides the body with a period of adjustment *en route* to the resting state. This lighter activity should continue until such time as breathing and heart rate approach normal values. It is then recommended that static stretching exercises be carried out whilst the muscle temperature is still raised. The combination of these activities (cool-down) is considered to:

1. aid muscular relaxation;
2. promote the removal of metabolic waste products from the muscles;
3. reduce muscle soreness.

Monitoring Exercise Intensity

It is important to realise that for each of us, according to our age and our recent history of activity, there is a safe and optimal intensity at which we should exercise. This is not a static value or threshold, but is dynamic and should reflect changes in our patterns of activity (or inactivity, whichever the case may be) as well as the ageing process. The assessment of exercise intensity is an especially important aspect for aerobic exercise. This is the case since the benefits of this type of activity are dependent upon individuals exercising within prescribed target zones. The target zone is the level of activity at which there is sufficient physiological stress to condition the muscles and cardiorespiratory system in order to achieve improved fitness.

For aerobic exercise these target zones have been constructed to incorporate upper and lower thresholds of exercise intensity for each individual, according to age and relative fitness (*see* tables on pages 19 and 20). The most commonly employed means of assessing the intensity of aerobic exercise is by monitoring of the exercise heart rate (pulse). Whilst

'Beginners' Target Heart Rate Zones (60–75% HRR)

Resting heart rate	[Age]										
	15–19	20–24	25–29	30–34	35–39	40–44	45–49	50–54	55–59	60–64	65–69
45–49	141–164	138–161	135–157	132–153	129–149	126–146	123–142	120–138	117–134	114–131	111–127
50–54	143–166	140–162	137–158	134–154	131–151	128–147	125–143	122–139	119–136	116–132	113–128
55–59	145–167	142–163	139–159	136–155	133–152	130–148	127–144	124–141	121–137	118–133	115–129
60–64	147–168	144–164	141–161	138–157	135–153	132–149	129–146	126–142	123–138	120–134	117–131
65–69	149–169	146–166	143–162	140–158	137–154	134–151	131–147	128–143	125–139	122–136	119–132
70–74	151–171	148–167	145–163	142–159	139–156	136–152	133–148	130–144	127–141	124–137	121–133
75–79	153–172	150–168	147–164	144–161	141–157	138–153	135–149	132–146	129–142	126–138	123–134
80–84	155–173	152–169	149–166	146–162	143–158	140–154	137–151	134–147	131–143	128–139	125–136
85–89	157–174	154–171	151–167	148–163	145–159	142–156	139–152	136–148	133–143	130–141	127–137

Monitoring exercise intensity for aerobic exercise: targets for beginners.

19

'Advanced' Target Heart Rate Zones (75–90% HRR)

Resting heart rate	[Age]										
	15–19	20–24	25–29	30–34	35–39	40–44	45–49	50–54	55–59	60–64	65–69
45–49	164–187	161–183	157–178	153–174	149–169	146–165	142–160	138–156	134–151	131–147	127–142
50–54	166–188	162–183	158–179	154–174	151–170	147–165	143–161	139–156	136–152	132–147	128–143
55–59	167–188	163–184	159–179	155–175	152–170	148–166	144–161	141–157	137–152	133–148	129–143
60–64	168–180	164–184	161–180	157–175	153–171	149–166	146–162	142–157	138–153	134–148	131–144
65–69	169–189	166–185	162–180	158–176	154–171	151–167	147–162	143–158	139–153	136–149	132–144
70–74	171–190	167–185	163–181	159–176	156–172	152–167	148–163	144–158	141–154	137–149	133–145
75–79	172–190	168–186	164–181	161–177	157–172	153–168	149–163	146–159	142–154	138–150	134–145
80–84	173–191	169–186	166–182	162–177	158–173	154–168	151–164	147–159	143–155	139–150	136–146
85–89	174–191	171–187	167–182	163–178	159–173	156–169	152–164	148–160	143–155	141–151	137–146

Monitoring exercise intensity for aerobic exercise: targets for those who exercise regularly.

ticated pulse-monitoring devices are now commercially available, this exercise parameter can be simply measured by manual palpation. This can be achieved as follows:

1. place the tips of your first two fingers lightly over one of the blood vessels in your neck (carotid arteries). These are located to the left or right of your windpipe (close to the Adam's apple). Alternatively, take the same two fingers and place them on the blood vessel which runs on the inside of your wrist (radial artery) just below the base of the thumb (*see* the illustrations on pages 48 and 49);
2. count the number of pulse beats for six seconds and then multiply by ten. This will give you a rough estimate of your exercise heart rate. It is important to appreciate that a miscount of only one beat in six seconds will result in an error of plus or minus ten beats per minute overall. Therefore it is recommended that you obtain a good deal of practice before you use this technique.

Calculating the Appropriate Intensity of Aerobic Exercise for You

To determine the intensity of aerobic exercise recommended for you it is first necessary to know two things:

1. your resting heart rate (RHR);
2. your maximal heart rate (MHR).

The former is easily measured by monitoring your pulse rate first thing in the morning, whilst still in bed. It is a good idea to record this RHR for a few mornings and then take the average value. The exact determination of the MHR requires you to undertake a maximal exercise test in a laboratory, during which time the exercise heart rate is recorded. There is, however, no need to panic at the thought of such rigours as the MHR can be estimated from the following formula:

220 – your age in years

Therefore the MHR for a 30-year old woman would be 220 – 30 = 190bpm.

So how do these two pieces of heart-rate

information combine to help us? The prescription of exercise intensity for aerobic exercise is most commonly prescribed by a formula employing a concept known as the heart-rate reserve (HRR). This refers to the difference between MHR and RHR. Therefore if we assume an RHR for our 30-year old woman of 70bpm her HRR would be calculated thus:

$$HRR = MHR - RHR$$
$$= 190 - 70$$
$$= 120bpm$$

As indicated above, both RHR and MHR are subject to change. RHR will generally decrease as a result of increased cardio-respiratory fitness, whilst MHR will decrease with increasing age (approximately at the rate of 1bpm per year).

Using the heart-rate data for our 30-year old woman as an example, one could calculate a specific intensity of exercise as follows:

$$60\% \ HRR = RHR + (0.6 \times HRR)$$
$$= 70 + (0.6 \times 120)$$
$$= 70 + 72$$
$$= 142bpm$$

However to eliminate the need for such calculations we have included two target heart rate zone tables (beginners and advanced). To use these all that is required is that upon determining your RHR (as outlined above) you locate this value in the relevant row, whilst at the same time locating your age in the appropriate column. Your target zone, showing upper and lower heart rate limits will be located where the RHR row and the age column intersect.

SOME TIPS TO HELP YOU STICK WITH YOUR HOME-BASED WORK-OUT

1. Draw up a plan of action and keep to it! Place it in a highly visible location – the fridge door is always a good place! Make the plan focus on creating a definite period of time each day for your exercise session.
2. Set yourself realistic goals. Aim for modest and gradual improvement.
3. Make your goals behavioural and not outcome-related. In other words set out to increase your duration/frequency/intensity of exercise rather than aim to lose x kilograms in y weeks. If you make the appropriate changes in behaviour the health-related benefits of exercise will look after themselves!
4. Each time you exercise, try to organise yourself so that you can exercise at a definite time and in a clearly defined space (your bedroom, for instance).
5. Try to enlist the support of your family and friends – better still get them to join in.
6. On days when you do not plan to exercise at home, try to get out and do some other form of exercise. Even simply going for a walk is a step in the direction of making activity part of your daily routine.
7. Always remember to warm up and cool down. Doing this will ensure that you reduce the possibility of injury.
8. Keep a record of your exercise progress, for example:

Week	1	3	5	7	9
Frequency	2	2	3	3	4
Duration (min)	20	25	25	30	30
Total exercise time (min)	40	50	75	90	120

9. Remember to assess continually your exercise programme – is it too easy? is it too hard? – and make the appropriate adjustments. Bear in mind that for the first three or four months you may find yourself making adjustments to the programme to increase the overload. Stick to the guidelines outlined above.

SECTION 1
THE WARM-UP

1 Before You Start

A WORD OF WARNING – AND ENCOURAGEMENT!

For some of you this may be the first exercise programme for some time. If you are over-weight, have a history of heart or lung disorders, asthma, diabetes, high blood pressure, bronchitis, bouts of dizziness, faint-ings, muscle or joint injury, or smoke, you should see your doctor before you start.

Do not let this precautionary advice deter you. Be positive about yourself and you *can* work out! Remember – there are three main rules. . . frequency, intensity and duration. Progress slowly, so as not to over-exert yourself; work at a comfortable pace. Work-ing out three times a week maintains your fitness level. Five times a week – and you will show great improvement.

Let's go to it!!

WHAT TO WEAR

What you work out on and what you work out in are very important. Exercising on inappro-priate surfaces and using improper footwear are known to cause lower body problems. The best type of floor to work out on is a sprung wooden floor, but few of us are fortunate enough to have one at home. Try not to work out on concrete or linoleum, both of which are very hard on the joints. These floors provide no 'give' and will not cushion your impact when you jump or hop. Before you start your work-out, make sure that the space is dry and clear of obstructions.

Footwear

Five years ago there were no shoes designed for aerobics. Now there are many. I choose Avia, but the choice is an individual one.

When selecting a shoe, look for a good fit and for comfort, trying on various models. A shoe should give you lateral support and stability. A good heel counter at the back of the shoe that holds the foot in place and that aids stability is also something to look for.

To get maximum wear out of your shoe, only wear them for aerobics – that way they will last longer, although you should examine your shoes regularly to see if they need replacing; badly worn shoes can cause in-juries. The top of the shoe may look fine, but remember to examine the amount of compres-sion in the cushioning layer.

Dress

Wear clothing that allows easy movement and enables you to see how your body is moving (your clothing should not be tight and restric-tive) – leotards and tights are probably best. You should also make sure that they are not made of heat retaining material such as sweat-suits which use plastic and so do not allow the skin to breathe. Layers of clothes are best so that as your muscles become warm a layer can be taken off once you are sufficiently warmed up. Very importantly, wear a leotard that makes you feel good about yourself and gives you confidence – so that you are raring to go.

The Achilles tendons and calf muscles can be kept warm during your work-out with leg-warmers (there is less chance of muscle strain when they are warm).

CONVENIENCE

Exercising at home is convenient. Set aside one hour a day (or every other day) for you – just you. Make it a priority in your daily schedule and I guarantee it will become part of your lifestyle.

When exercising, use a mirror to work in front of whenever you can. In this way you can observe your techniques, particularly looking at your knees, ankles, toes, hips, back and neck and can maintain a good body alignment throughout your work-out.

SAFETY

Never sacrifice speed for safety. When running on the spot, land on the ball of the foot followed by the heel and when travelling across the floor, land on the heel, followed by the ball of the foot. For the first few weeks, keep your work-out at a very low level; a good, long warm-up (15–20 minutes), a short aerobic section, a short strength section and a long stretch and relaxation section, perhaps totalling one hour will probably suffice. As the weeks go on, aerobic and strength sections can increase, always remembering to work within your own limitations. You must also be patient; fitness cannot be achieved overnight. Work out regularly, at least three times a week to maintain any level of fitness and five times a week to increase your level of fitness. Remember, build up gradually and do not do too much too soon; muscles, joints, bones, ligaments and tendons all need to be eased into activity safely, gradually and effectively.

NON-IMPACT MOVEMENT

Points to Remember

1. To reduce stress to the lower body, you should incorporate non-impact moves, keeping high-impact moves in your aerobics (cardiovascular) section.
2. Non-impact movement reduces the force of impact of the foot hitting the floor. One foot should remain on the floor at all times; there should be no jumping or hopping when doing a move.
3. When travelling to the side, forwards and backwards, keep your leg movements close to the floor and your knees slightly bent.
4. Avoid changing directions rapidly; do a 'transition move' in place before changing direction.
5. Control your movements at all times and avoid swinging the weights. Keep the elbow joints 'soft'.
6. Your knees should be bent over your toes during movements; be careful in lateral movements that your knees do not turn in.
7. Be aware of your target zone (see Introduction) and how to alter your heart rate or intensity. For example, to reduce your intensity, limit your range of motion in some movements or eliminate arm movements altogether.
8. Intensity can also be reduced by travelling less across the floor or by smaller knee lifts and smaller kicks.
9. Remember, especially when working out with a friend, a move that is good for someone else is not necessarily good for you.
10. Listen to your body, find the exercises that best suit you and use them to your advantage.
11. After several weeks, when the moves become easier, a one-pound (half-kilogram) weight can be added to increase the intensity of your exercise.
12. Be aware of how you use your arms.

25

THE SELECTION OF MUSIC

Points to Remember

1. Good music is a great motivator to working out. It also provides the timing and speed for your exercise movements.
2. Before you start to work out, plan your programmes, select your music carefully and perhaps put together a tape. Select music that is *fun*. A tempo of 100–120 beats per minute is frequently used for warming up, while the aerobic components are generally performed at a tempo of 130–160 beats per minute and strength work at 110–130 beats per minute – this is a good, steady beat. Stretch and relaxation should be done to music of 100–110 beats per minute.
3. The warm-up music needs to be 'beaty' but comfortable and not too fast.
4. The aerobic music needs to be 'beaty' but not too slow.
5. The strength-work music must not be too fast; the right tempo will allow you to move under control.
6. The stretch music needs to be slow and relaxing.
7. Select movement patterns that fit each segment of your music. Try to repeat your steps in a regular series of four or eight counts with smooth transitions.
8. Avoid music that is too fast during the aerobic content and which forces you to remain on the balls of your feet for extended periods of time.
9. After you have been working out with music regularly, you will feel more confident and perhaps want to use a freer and more spontaneous method which requires less preparation.
10. Always bear in mind safety and effectiveness.

SAFETY, EFFECTIVENESS

1. Avoid hyperextension of any joints.
2. Stay off the balls of your feet.
3. Bend your knees, especially on landing.
4. Avoid flailing limbs.
5. Do not overwork.
6. Breathe regularly.
7. Try to avoid lateral moves.
8. Do not 'bounce' when stretching.
9. Work under control.
10. Do not repeat a move more than four times on one leg, but rather alternate.

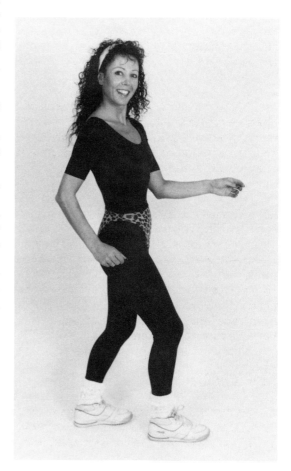

THE TOTAL WORK-OUT

This work-out programme contains every possible aspect of your home-based aerobics exercises, including:

1. warm-up (mobility, stretching and pulse-raiser);
2. cardiovascular fitness;
3. muscle strength;
4. muscle endurance;
5. motor fitness;
6. agility;
7. power;
8. balance;
9. reaction time;
10. speed;
11. co-ordination;
12. flexibility;
13. relaxation.

Another important thing to remember is that you do not need to be an athlete in order to enjoy participating in regular exercise. However there are some basic points which you should bear in mind when you embark upon your aerobic programme:

1. set realistic goals;
2. work out with a friend;
3. do not compete;
4. have a positive attitude towards fitness and health;
5. practise your skills;
6. do not worry about ability;
7. do not be a weekend-only athlete;
8. have fun, enjoy exercise.

POSTURE

The photograph on this page shows the ideal postural alignment; keep your head vertical, feel as if you are lengthening your neck. Bring your chin slightly in towards your neck,

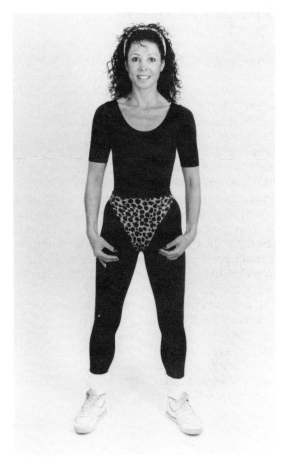

pressing your shoulders back and down and keeping them relaxed. Your rib-cage is directly over your pelvis (neither forward nor back) which is 'resting' over your hips and should not be tipped forward or backward.

Your back, too, should be in a relaxed, vertical line and your knees should be over your toes with the weight just behind the balls of your feet – which face straight ahead. You should unlock your knees to enable your entire body to be balanced and to move efficiently, freely and safely. Ensure that you breathe comfortably.

THE FIRST WEEK

The FITT principle (frequency, intensity, time, type) should always be borne in mind when starting an exercise programme. Accordingly, you must decide how often, how hard, when and what sort of exercise you will perform.

The intensity at which you work out should always be comfortable for you. If you are not particularly fit, your heart rate will be raised very quickly, so always take things easy initially; progresssion must be gradual.

The golden rule here is not to do too much too soon. Take at least fifteen minutes for your warm-up and about five to eight minutes for your aerobic work-out, which should alternate between high and low intensity. You may not want to exercise your arms during the first week as this can elevate your pulse too much; it may therefore be safer in your first few days not to work your arms. After three or four weeks, when you feel your work-out getting easier and you need more of a challenge, slowly begin to increase your pace – either by taking bigger steps or by doing more work involving raising your arms above your head. If, however, you feel winded at any time, you should reduce the intensity at which you are working, perhaps simply marching on the spot for a few moments.

Strength Work for the Upper and Lower Body

In the early stages of your work-out, do not use bands or weights. Simply start by doing about two sets of eight repetitions of various exercises, working for about ten or so minutes – with rests if and when you need them.

As you progress and the exercises become easier, start to increase the workload by doing greater numbers of sets and repetitions. Once you feel you are ready, you should introduce weights or bands – returning to the beginning again so far as sets and repetitions are concerned. Adding resistance greatly increases the difficulty of these exercises and you will fatigue much more quickly.

Again as you practice, gradually add sets and repetitions and reduce the number of rest periods. By the ten or twelfth week you should have increased your session from ten to about fifteen or twenty minutes. One other point to mention is that you should always alternate the muscle groups that you exercise. Great care is called for here since it is easy to alter the exercise but still work the same muscles.

To begin, it is best to exercise two or three times a week, taking about forty-five minutes for each work-out. Gradually increase this to four or five times a week, but remember not to do too much too soon.

Summary

The first week is essentially a prolonged warm-up session of short, low-intensity aerobic exercises. It may also include a brief strength section, but without weights or bands, as well as long sections devoted to stretching and relaxation. By the fifth or sixth week, the warm-up will be a little shorter – as will the stretch and relaxation sections – with the aerobic and strength work becoming correspondingly longer. After fifteen or twenty weeks you will probably have progressed to three or more sessions a week (with a total work-out time of over an hour). As you would expect, once again the stretch and relaxation periods are shorter – perhaps eight or ten minutes out of a total of twenty or more minutes. Strength work will form a greater proportion of the work-out than before; there should be few if any rest periods.

If you are always aware of the FITT principle, regularly sip water, wear good shoes, work on a good surface and have great, motivating music, you can't go wrong.

2 Mobility and Pulse-raising

EXERCISE 1

Shoulder Rolls

Stand with your legs apart, firm stomach, knees slightly bent and arms loosely to your side. Extend your neck up in a long vertical line and keep your head straight. Your ears should be directly above your shoulders and your jaw relaxed. Slowly, for the count of four, bring your shoulders up and then slowly pull them back and down for four. Follow this with eight back and eight forward.

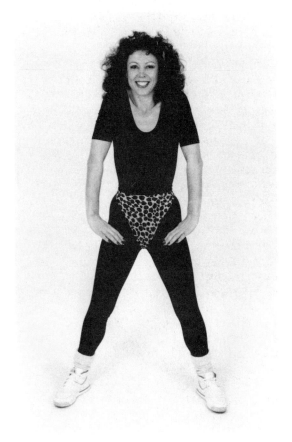

EXERCISE 2

Shoulder Lifts

Your feet should be hip-distance apart and your knees bent. Lift your shoulders up and back and then lower them slowly. Do two sets of eight and repeat. Then do two sets of eight forward.

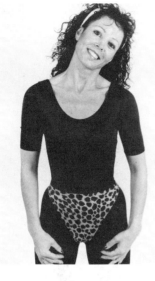

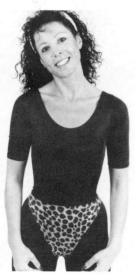

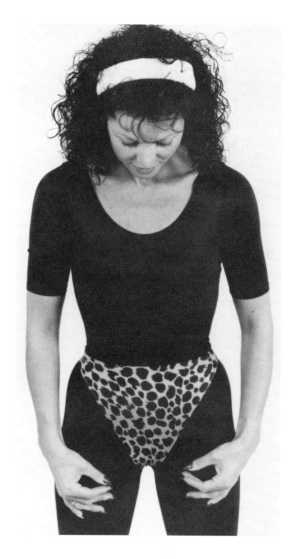

EXERCISE 4

Chin Down

Push your chin towards your chest and then up again. Repeat this four times. Do *not* bend your neck backwards and ensure that you breathe throughout the movement.

EXERCISE 3

Head Tilts

With relaxed shoulders and slightly bent knees, press your left ear down towards your left shoulder. Then return to the centre before pressing your other ear towards your right shoulder. Repeat to left and right four times each.

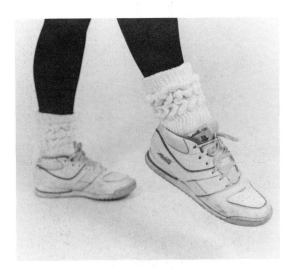

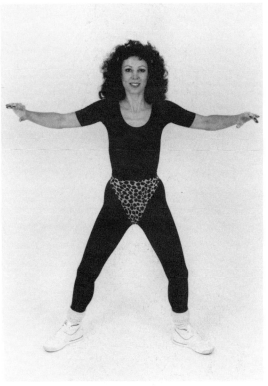

EXERCISE 5

Warming up the Ankle

Stand with the correct posture as shown on page 27. Lift your right leg off the floor and bend your knees. Slowly lift your right foot up towards the lower leg, flex for two counts and lower towards the floor. Repeat this four times.

Slowly, for two counts, move the toe to the right corner and then to the left. Repeat this four times.

Rotate the ankle slowly through a complete range of motion clockwise for the count of four and anti-clockwise for the count of four. Do this four times and change legs.

EXERCISE 6

Knee Bends

With your feet just over hip-distance apart and in a comfortable stance place your knees directly above your ankles which are pointing out, in the same direction as your toes. Slowly, and with control, flex your knee joint and extend it in a straight line. Do not move your bottom lower than your knees as this puts excessive pressue on the knees and do not let your knees roll inwards as they bend. Your hips should be directly under your shoulders and your back in a straight line. Lift your rib-cage and relax your shoulders. Perform one set of eight.

31

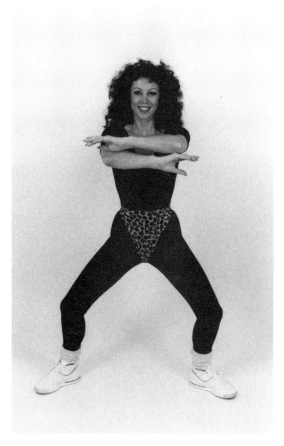

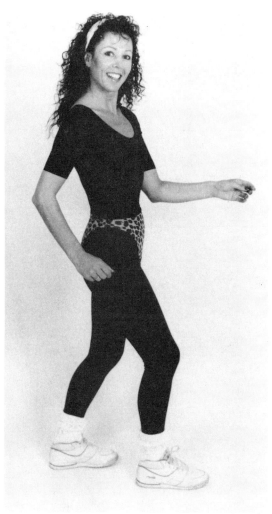

EXERCISE 7

Knee Bends with Arms

Bend slowly at the knees in a controlled manner and then lift the arms to shoulder height, gently bringing them across your chest and returning them to the starting position in line with the shoulder. You should press your shoulder-blades together and keep your elbows 'soft'. Take care not to throw your arms back – which can cause stress to the shoulder joint and arching of the back. Breathe regularly and perform one set of eight.

EXERCISE 8

Forward Walks

Walk forwards – one, two, three, four – pressing down on your heels. Then walk backwards – one, two, three, four – again pressing down on your heels. Repeat four times in each direction.

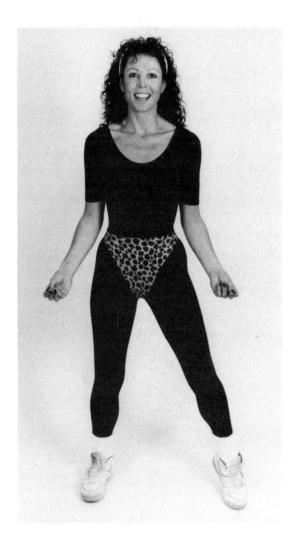

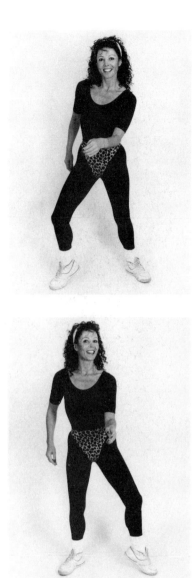

EXERCISE 9

While being aware of your posture and with slightly bent knees and a straight back, perform a side dig-step to the left, the right, the left, the right and so on. Keep your arms into your waist and 'snap' your hands down and up for sixteen counts, then out to the side for sixteen counts and finally alternate the arms for a total of sixteen counts.

EXERCISE 10

For this move, you need to take slightly bigger steps as you perform a diagonal lunge to the right. Move your right toe with a bent knee and then press your heel to the floor. Perform this sixteen times and repeat to the left. Then walk forwards and backwards diagonally to the left and to the right four times each.

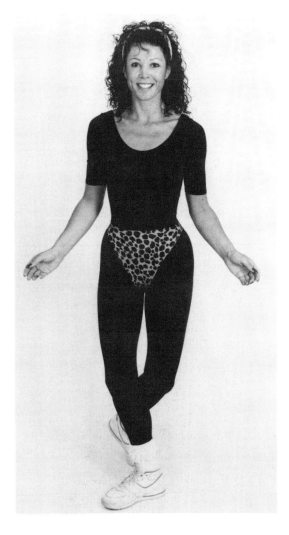

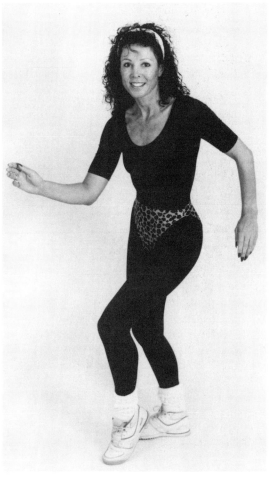

EXERCISE 12

Side Walks

Walk to the right – one, two, three, four – and on four lift your knee and turn. Then walk to the left – one, two, three, four – and on four lift your knee again. Repeat four times in each direction.

EXERCISE 11

The Grapevine

Step to the side on the right foot and then bring your left foot across behind your right foot – before moving it back to the left and moving your right behind your left. Repeat sixteen times.

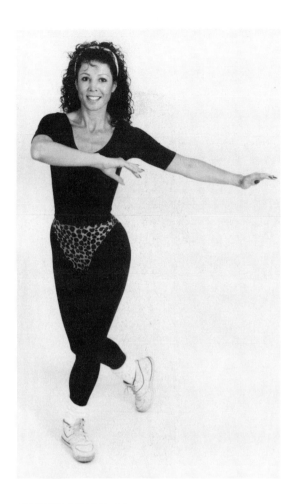

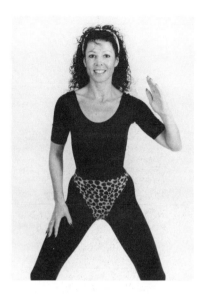

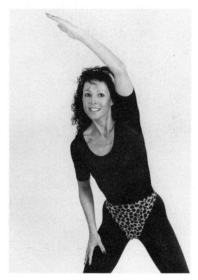

EXERCISE 13

Step Touches

Step left and touch the floor behind with your right foot, then step right and touch the floor behind with your left foot. Swing your arm across your chest as shown for each direction. Perform two sets of eight and then repeat, incorporating a clap with the same movement of the feet.

EXERCISE 14

Lifts

Bend your knees and on the rise reach up with one arm and then the other. Your movement should flow and not be jerky. Breathe comfortably, and watch your posture. Perform to the right and left a total of sixteen times.

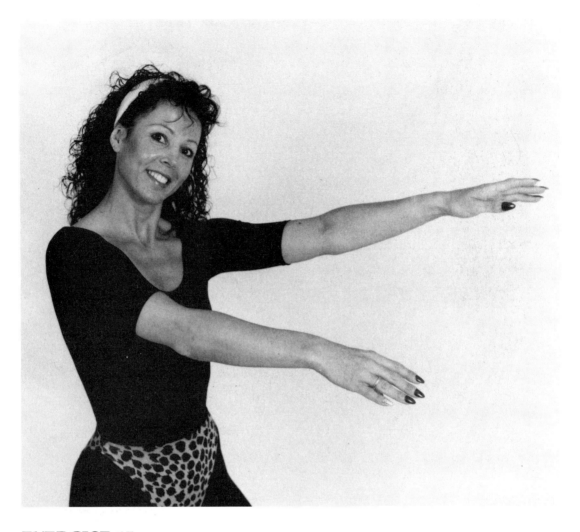

EXERCISE 15

Arm Sweeps

Stand with your feet just over hip-distance apart (this is a good, wide supporting base). Bend your knees directly over your ankles, making sure that they do not roll inwards. The arms start in a horizontal position, facing away from your body. As the knees bend, bring one arm down and around in front of your body in a very controlled manner to meet the other arm. Perform two sets of eight.

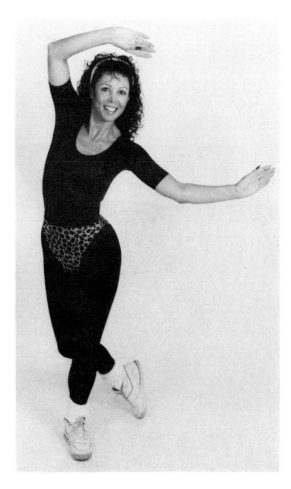 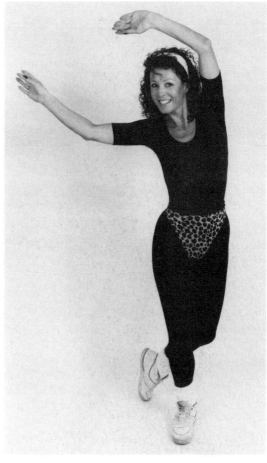

EXERCISE 16

Step Touch

Stand with your feet apart and your arms at shoulder height. Step and touch back with the right foot, bringing both arms up and over to one side, then step and touch back with your left foot taking your arms to the other side. Do not exaggerate this move and keep it under control, ensuring that at all times your arms are kept to the front of your body. You should pull in your stomach – but not arch your back, pointing your knees in the same direction as your toes. Perform two sets of eight.

37

3 Preparatory Stretches

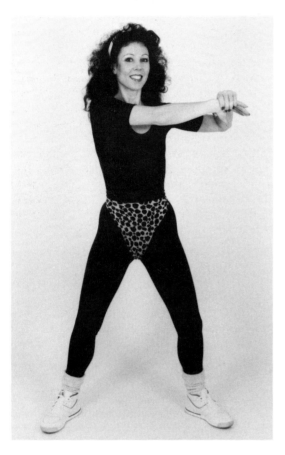

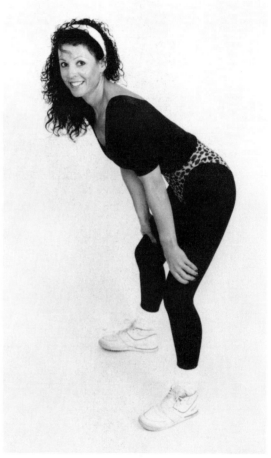

EXERCISE 17

Shoulder Stretch

Bring your right arm across your chest and gently pull it towards your chest with your left hand, feeling slight pressure (but not pain) in your shoulder. Hold for about eight seconds and repeat with the other arm.

EXERCISE 18

Lower Back Stretch

Put your hands on your knees to support the upper body and then curve the lower back by using the abdominal muscles to produce a 'pelvic tilt'.

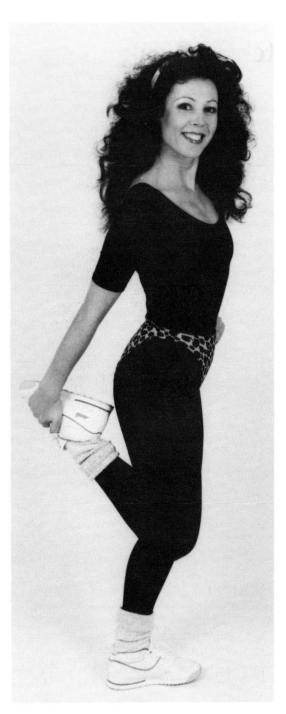

EXERCISE 19

The Thighs

Make sure you keep a good position while performing this exercise. Keep your body upright with your pelvis also in an upright, 'neutral' position, your back in a straight line and your shoulders in a relaxed position. Lift one leg towards your bottom and then grasp hold of the foot and gently pull it towards your buttocks. Make sure you do not squeeze the knee by forcing your foot too high as this can cause the knee to be over-strained (remember, stretching is particular to each individual; what one person can safely do might prove dangerous for another). You should also ensure that your knee points down towards the floor and that you bend your supporting leg slightly. Hold for about eight seconds before changing legs.

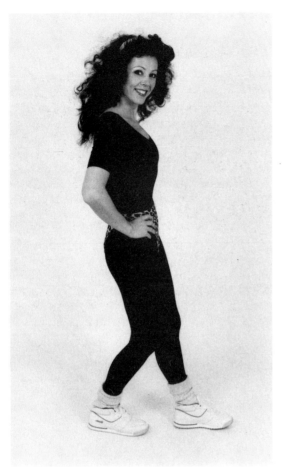

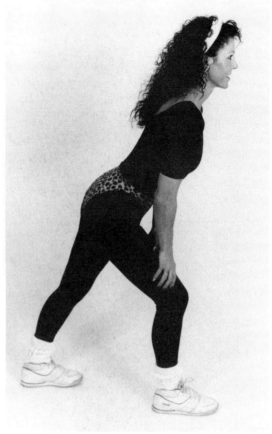

EXERCISE 20

Calf and Ankle Stretch

Stand in an upright position, one leg forward, one leg back, with your heels flat on the floor and your toes straight ahead. Transfer your weight slightly backwards over your back heel and then slowly, and with control, bend your back knee. Slight tension should be felt in the lower calf and the back of the heel. Hold for a count of eight and then straighten the knee. Repeat with the other leg.

EXERCISE 21

Calf and Hip Stretch

Stand as instructed at the beginning of Exercise 20. Bend your front knee and move body-weight forward slightly (the knee should be directly over the ankle, not beyond the toes). Your back leg extends backwards, the heel pressed to the floor and your abdominal muscles tight. Then push the hip above the back leg forward to stretch your hip flexors, keeping the body in a straight line from the head to the back heel. Hold for eight counts.

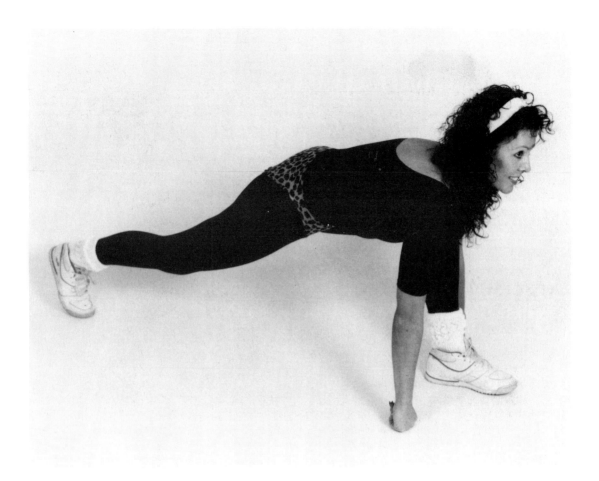

EXERCISE 22

Runner's Lunge

Adopt the starting position shown above. Bend your front knee, but again not beyond your toes. Place your hands on the floor with your back leg extended out as far as possible behind you. Gently press your hips down towards the floor (without bouncing – this is a static stretch). Hold for eight counts.

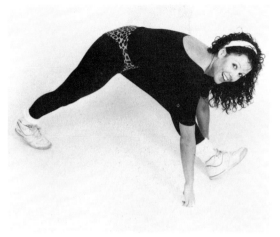

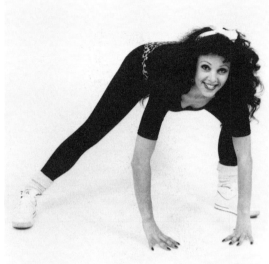

EXERCISE 23

The Hamstring Stretch

Adopt the same position as shown in Exercise 22 and then transfer your weight back, with a 'soft' knee joint and a firm stomach. Lift the toes of your front foot up and down for eight counts and try to press your back heel down before returning to the position of the runner's lunge for eight counts. Change legs and repeat.

EXERCISE 24

The Inner Thigh

Stand upright with your left knee bent and your right leg extended to the side. Lower the upper body slowly towards the floor and place your hands on the floor to support your body and take the pressure off your knees, keeping your heels down. Be careful not to lock the knee of your extended leg. Then move your body slowly over to one side, holding this position for eight seconds before changing sides. To come up, shift your upper body towards your bent knee in order to maintain balance and to enable you to rise safely. The stretch should be felt on the inner thigh and the groin.

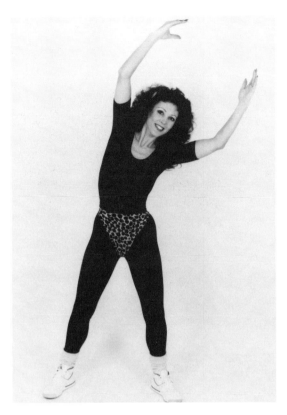

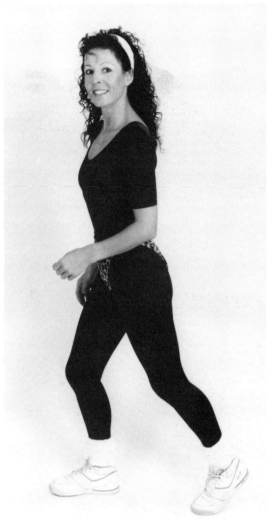

EXERCISE 25

The Rib-cage

Place your feet just over hip-distance apart. Bend your knees slightly and keep your back straight (*not* arched). Then lift your arms high above your head, but keeping your shoulder-blades down and relaxed and with your elbows slightly bent. This stretch is felt in the lower part of the ribs and should be held for about eight seconds. Slowly, and with control, reach left towards the top corner of the room and hold this position for another eight seconds (this stretch will be felt on your left side). Return to the central position using your side muscles and stretch to the other side and hold for a further eight seconds before returning to the centre and slowly lowering your arms.

EXERCISE 26

Walking around the Room

If you have the space, walk fairly quickly around the room. Start to increase the length of your steps and pump your arms more vigorously to elevate your pulse. Always walk in the opposite direction equally to counteract lateral stress.

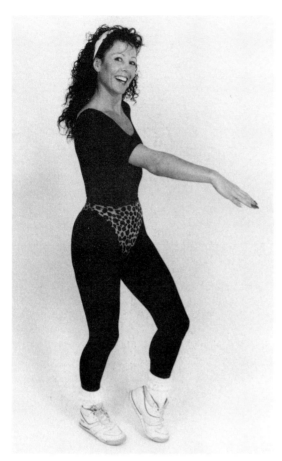 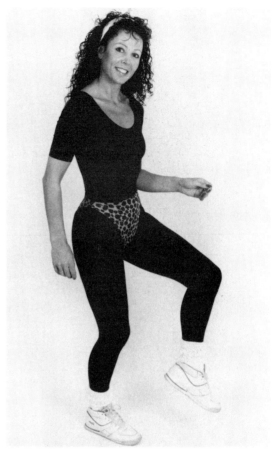

EXERCISE 27

Moving Backwards and Forwards with a Knee Lift

Move in time – one, two, three – lifting your knee slightly each time. Your knees should be relaxed and directly above your toes and your stomach should be firm. Lift your arms alternately and under control, but move them further than you have moved your knees. Breathe regularly and perform the exercise four times going forwards and four times going backwards. Repeat this twice.

44

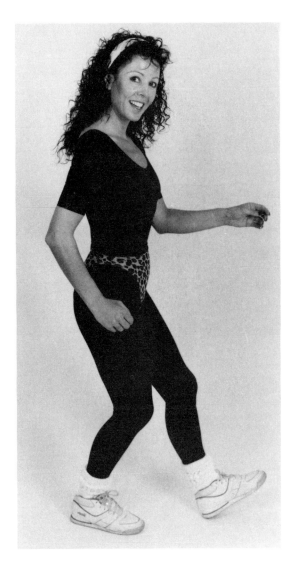

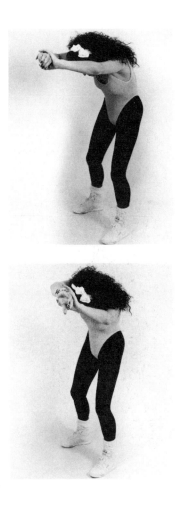

EXERCISE 29

Back and Side Stretch

Stand with your feet shoulder-width apart, your knees bent, your pelvis in a neutral position and your back rounded. Raise your arms above your head and grasp your wrist with your other hand; then gently pull your arm sideways to stretch one side of your body. Simultaneously, tuck your pelvis in and relax your lower spine – then hold the stretch before returning to the starting position and repeating on the other side. You should stretch for about eight seconds before changing sides.

EXERCISE 28

As for the previous exercise, except that on the fourth count, plant your heel firmly on to the floor. Pump your arms and repeat as directed in Exercise 27.

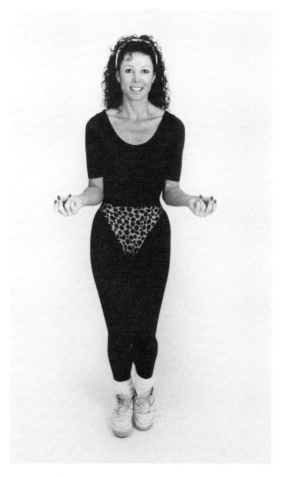

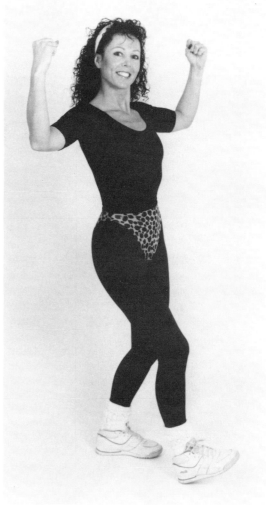

EXERCISE 30

Step to the side with one foot, knees bent, and then bring the other foot to it – step touch, step touch – making the movement fluid and taking the arms side to side at the same time. You can add a variation by moving forwards and backwards and by changing the arm movements as you wish. Start to increase your intensity by making larger movements side to side, not forgetting to check for good body control and alignment throughout.

EXERCISE 31

Bicep Curl with Heel Press

Move your arms up to shoulder height, with your elbows bent. Then curl your fists in towards your shoulders, simultaneously pressing your heels down alternately. Aim to maintain good posture throughout.

SECTION 2
THE WORK-OUT

1 The Aerobics Programme

THE AEROBIC COMPONENT

There are various moves to perform throughout this running section – change them around as you wish but do not do more than eight repetitions on one leg. You should breathe regularly throughout the work-out so that there is a good supply of oxygen for the working muscles. As you land on the ball of your foot, try to make sure you bring your heel down on to the floor to absorb the stress and lessen the pressure on the front of your leg. Whenever possible, your running movements should be in units of four, forwards, backwards or diagonally – you should also avoid locking your knees and aim to keep them 'soft' – supple and flexible.

Start at a very low level and increase the intensity gently and comfortably, and then, towards the end of aerobic session, gradually reduce intensity. During the session you should include both high and low intensity non-impact moves – and at the end, having reduced the intensity of your work-out, you should keep the body moving for at least five minutes to allow your pulse rate to return to normal. You should be able to take your pulse yourself – and the next two illustrations below show where you should place your fingers in order to feel your pulse at your wrist (the radial artery) and at your neck (the carotid artery). Start the work-out slowly by low-intensity jogging on the spot (always being aware of your target heart rate). Increase your jogging to slightly bigger steps but do

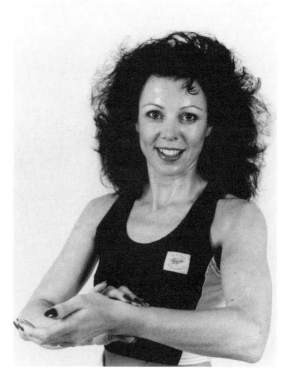

This illustration shows where you should take your pulse on your wrist (the radial artery).

not swing your arms. Gradually increase the work-load by moving your arms and taking bigger steps. If at any time the intensity becomes too great, reduce your arm and leg movements or travel less across the floor.

Use the walk–run method, remembering to make good, safe, controlled movements. A

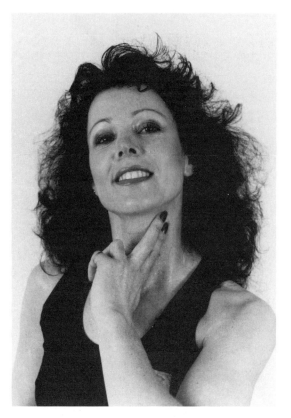

Where to take your pulse on your neck (the carotid artery).

gradual increase in duration and good foot-wear are also both essential to avoid musculo-skeletal injury. You may find the work-out difficult at first, but as you perform it regularly, so you will build up your stamina.

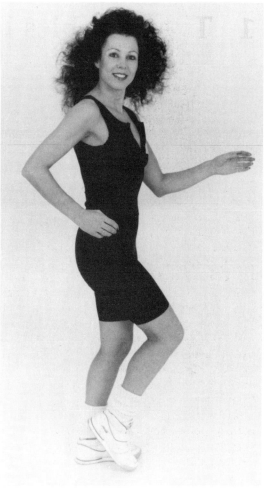

EXERCISE 32

Jog quite slowly on the spot for 32 counts, pressing your heels down and keeping the feet close to the floor for a low-impact jog. The supporting knee should be slightly flexed and when lifting the knee, move it up and forward. After about two or three minutes begin to combine arm movements, pumping your arms forward and backward to increase the intensity.

49

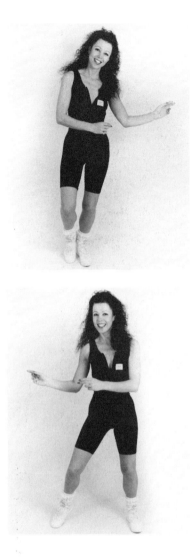

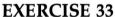

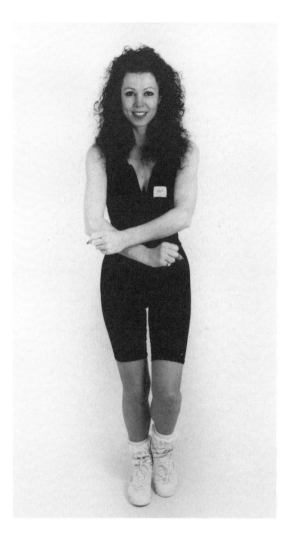

EXERCISE 33

Chassé

Glide forwards (chassé) three steps – one, two, three – the right foot steps forward, the left then moves up behind it and the right foot steps forward again on three. The movement should be kept smooth. When moving to the side, the right foot glides to one side, the left moves beside it and, on three, the right slides once again to the side.

EXERCISE 34

Stand with your knees slightly bent and your arms crossed in front of your body. With control, move your leg to the side and touch the floor with the heel, your toes pointing to the ceiling. At the same time, lift your arms up to shoulder level (but no further) then return to the starting position and repeat eight times on each leg.

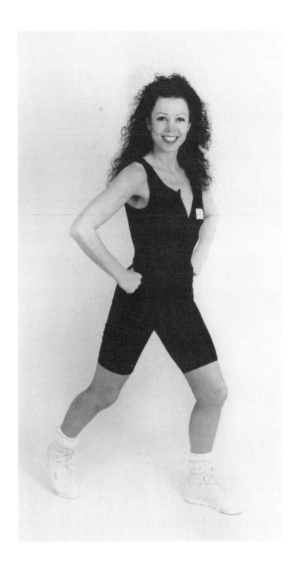

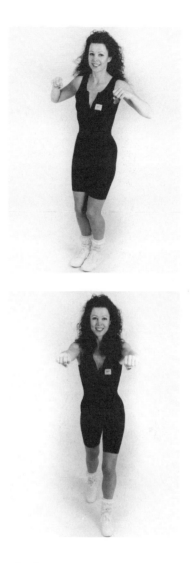

EXERCISE 35

Stand with your feet hip-width apart and your knees slightly bent. Bend your arms with your elbows behind your torso, keeping your knees bent and then take a step back with your right foot. At the same time extend your forearms behind your torso without moving your elbow (taking care not to lock the elbow joints). Finally, bring your leg forward and return the forearms to the starting position. Repeat eight times.

EXERCISE 36

Start with your legs hip-distance apart, your knees slightly bent and your shoulders relaxed. Bend your arms and place your hands in front of your shoulders, moving your right foot back and tapping with the ball of your foot. At the same time straighten your arms in front of the chest and bring your hands back to your shoulders as your legs return to the starting position. Repeat on the other leg and perform sixteen times.

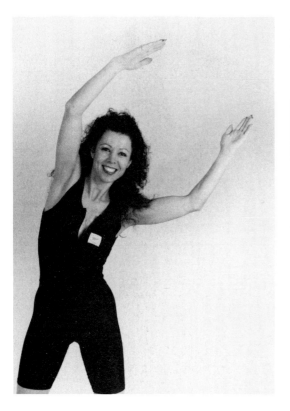

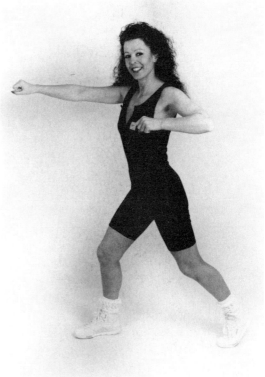

EXERCISE 37

With slightly bended knees slowly lift up your arms and shift your weight to your right, straightening your left leg. At the same time, push both your arms to the upper right diagonal and then return to the starting position before changing to the other side. Each push from one side to the other counts as one repetition and you should perform a total of eight pushes. Do not forget to exhale on effort (as you move your arms).

EXERCISE 38

Lunge with a Punch

Stand with your feet together then jump to one side and lunge with your weight distributed evenly over both feet, keeping your hips and shoulders square and taking care not to twist your body as you land. Then punch one arm straight out in front of you – without locking your elbow. Do a total of about sixteen lunges.

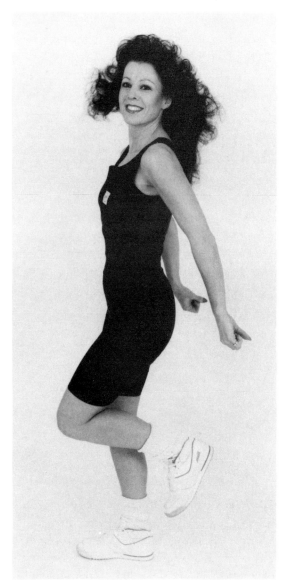
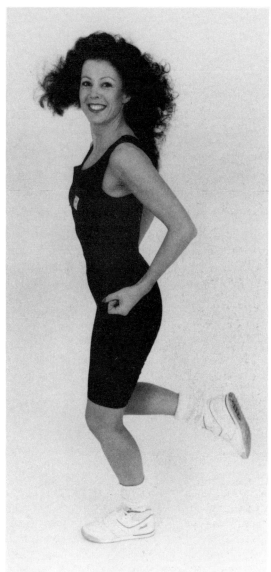

EXERCISE 39

Jog while Pumping your Arms Backwards

Press back your elbows and curl your fore-arms up towards your chest while jogging. You should take care not to let your elbows swing forwards. As you kick, lift your heels as high as possible towards your buttocks. Move forwards for four counts – and then back for four.

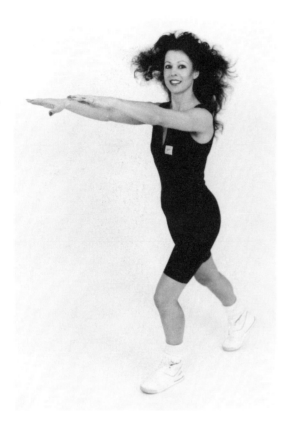

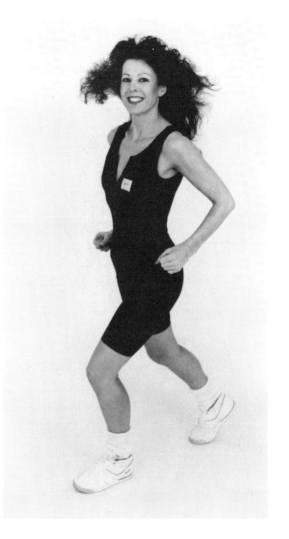

EXERCISE 40

Start with your feet together and your arms relaxed by your sides. Lunge, alternating your forward leg ensuring that the knee of your front leg does not extend beyond your toes and that your shoulders are relaxed. Bend your arms down towards your waist and then extend them in front of your chest. Exhale as you thrust out your arms. Keep the heel of your front leg flat on the floor when landing.

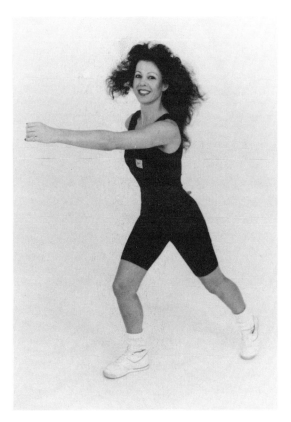 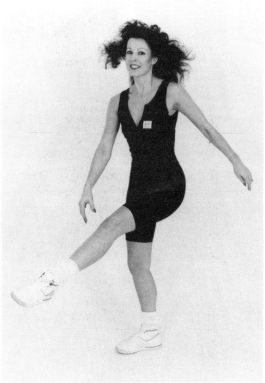

EXERCISE 41

Shoot your left leg back and your right arm forward, then move your right leg back and your left arm forward in a pumping action, keeping your chest high.

EXERCISE 42

Keeping your arms and legs low to begin with, kick your right leg and then your left with the opposite arm swinging forwards while the other arm swings back. You should lift your leg only as far as is comfortable and avoid high kicking.

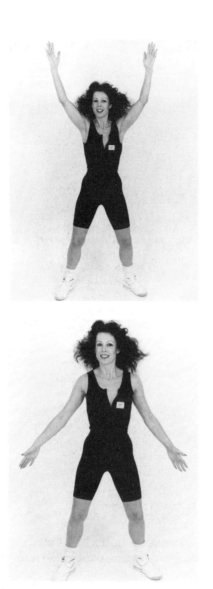

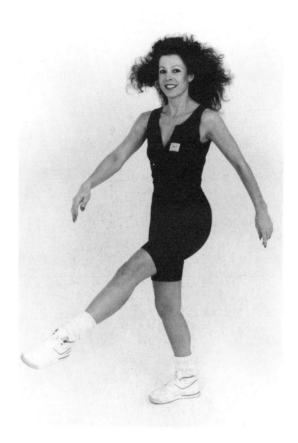

EXERCISE 43

Jumping Jacks

Start with your feet shoulder-width apart, your knees bent and your arms raised above your head. Jump, bringing your feet together and your arms down to the side of your body. As you land you should bend your knees slightly and *not* arch your back.

EXERCISE 44

Kicks

As for Exercise 42 but slowly increase intensity by raising your arms and legs higher, kicking first your right and then your left leg. Try to lift your thigh without momentum – do not swing your leg. Keep your back straight and do not move your chest towards your knee. Your heel should land on the floor with each jump and you should breathe regularly. You can start to travel after a while, perhaps having a programme which will involve you kicking four times to the right, turning and travelling four counts to the left.

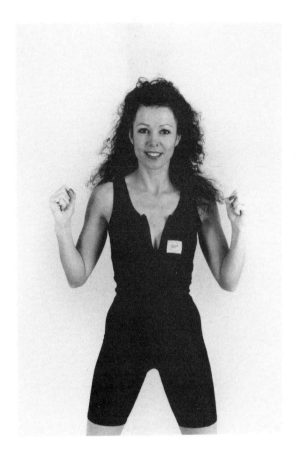

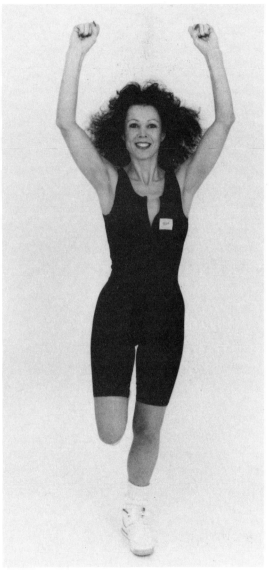

EXERCISE 45

Jog with Overhead Press

Jog on the spot, keeping your back straight and your rib-cage lifted. Land on the ball of your foot – quickly followed by your heels and bending your knees on landing. Your arms are pressed above your head and lowered to waist level, bending them at the elbow. Do two sets of eight and then travel forward for four counts and backward for four. You can also change the exercise slightly by landing on your heel first – and then your toes.

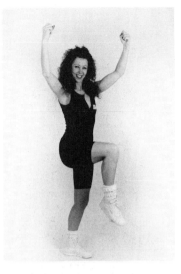

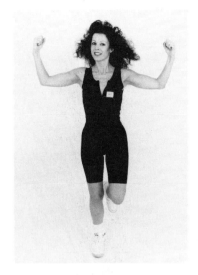

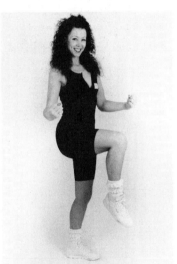

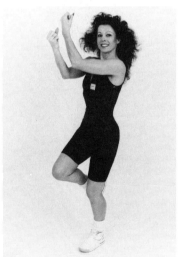

EXERCISE 46

Knee Lifts

Stand with your back straight, your knees bent above your toes and your arms extended overhead. Under control, pull your arms down and at the same time lift your right knee in front of your body. Repeat standing on the other leg and perform eight lifts with each leg.

EXERCISE 47

Cross-overs

With your arms at shoulder height and pressing your elbows together, jog forward for four counts and back for four – again pressing your heels down and keeping your knees over your toes. Lift your elbows to chest height and cross in front. Perform two sets of eight.

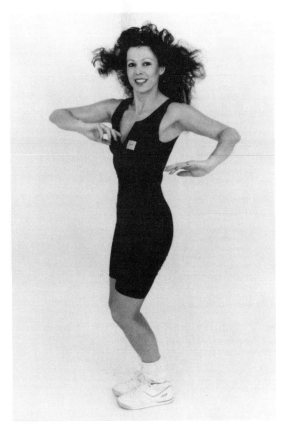

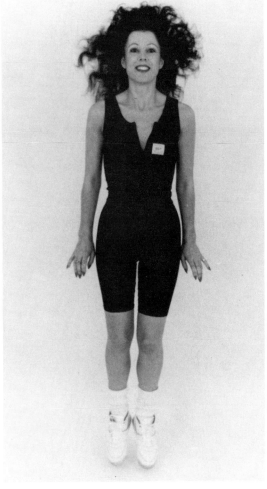

EXERCISE 48

Twist

Twist with your feet together, your heels on the floor, your knees bent (facing right) and your back straight. Lift your arms to chest height to the left and switch the twist, changing feet and arm positions and keeping your feet and knees together and your torso erect. There should be no arching of your back. Twist to the right for eight counts – then twist to the left for another eight counts. Jog on the spot, moving fists to your shoulders and your elbows up and down to the sides. Do this for eight counts to each side.

EXERCISE 49

Jump up and down on the spot, remembering to bend the knees and keeping your heels down on landing. Do this for one set of eight repetitions, then move one leg forward to touch the floor with your heel; your toes should face the ceiling and you should alternate your heels. Perform one set of eight, ensuring that your knees are kept supple, 'soft'.

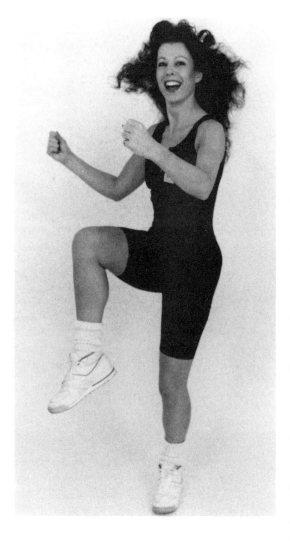

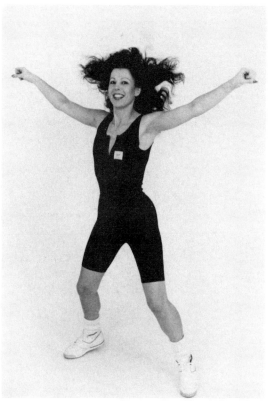

EXERCISE 51

Stand with your feet together and your hands by your side. Jump and move your feet so that they are shoulder-distance apart; then move your arms to shoulder height. Make sure that your knees bend on landing and that your elbow joints are 'soft'. Every movement should be done with control. Do one set of eight.

EXERCISE 50

In this exercise you must keep your knees up and your back straight. Lift your right knee up in front of your body while pulling your arms down. Keep your shoulders back and relaxed. Do eight, then jog forward for four counts, back for four and do eight more with your knees high. Repeat this sequence so that you perform two sets.

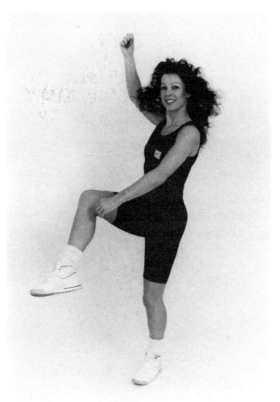
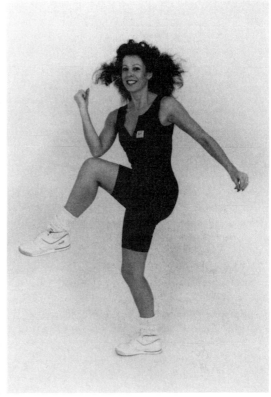

EXERCISE 52

Knee Lifts

Stand with your feet shoulder-width apart and your arms extended to the side. Keep your stomach tight and your back straight. Lift one knee diagonally across your body, bringing the elbow of the opposite arm in to your knee. Alternate the arm and leg – right, left, right, left. Perform two sets of eight movements (a movement means moving to the left and right). Breathe regularly.

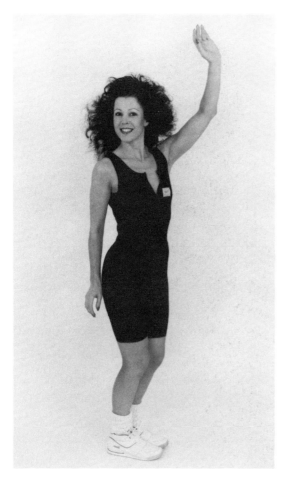 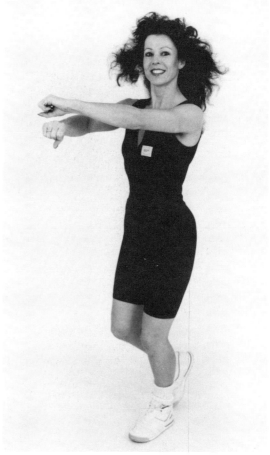

EXERCISE 53

Keep your feet together as you jump up and down and twist from side to side. Pump your arms up in turn, making sure that as you land your heels go down on the floor. Bend your knees, with your knees above your toes, your torso erect, your back straight and your pelvis tucked in. Do one set of eight and then repeat this exercise, adding to the work-load by bending your knees lower. Do one set of eight and then move your feet shoulder width apart and twist. Once again, do one set of eight.

EXERCISE 54

Vertical Scissors

Extend your arms in front of your body with your palms facing down and then 'scissor' your arms in front of your chest, moving one arm to the other. Do four sets of four using your right arm, four sets of four using your left and then, moving both arms towards each other, one set of eight to the front. In this exercise your feet are barely moving, so that your pulse does not become too high.

EXERCISE 55

Chest Crosses

First of all, raise your arms towards the ceiling, then move one hand in front of the other so that they each point towards a different corner of the ceiling. Then cross your arms at the elbow, still pointing towards the ceiling, alternating which is nearest your face – left, right, left, right – next, cross your arms actually in front of your face and alternate.

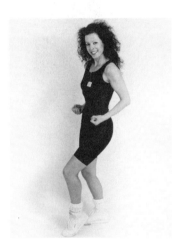

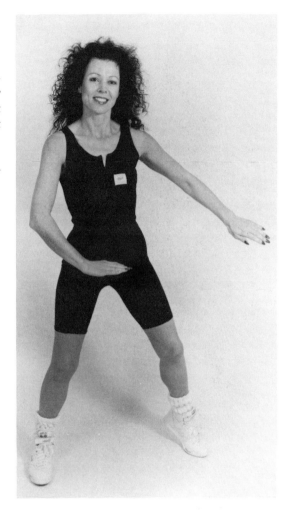

EXERCISE 56

Cool-down 1

By gradually reducing the intensity of your movements to a very low level, (slowly lower your arms and make smaller leg movements) you will reduce your heart rate towards resting levels and prevent excessive pooling of blood in your legs. You will also feel your breathing getting easier.

Walk forward three times, dig step on the fourth and then clap. Walk backwards three times, dig step on the fourth and clap twice. Do the same movement to the side, both left and right, clapping first once, then twice.

EXERCISE 57

Lunge

You should not jump during this low-intensity exercise. Turn to the right, bend your left knee and step forward with your right foot to form the lunge position. Straighten your left arm and press the right towards the floor with a bent elbow (as shown). Repeat the exercise, turning to the left and repeat in all sixteen times.

63

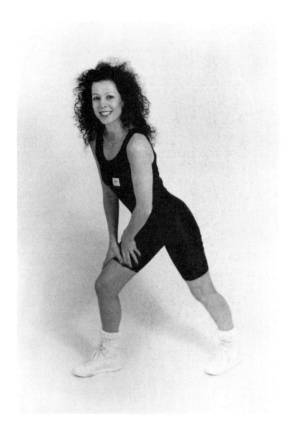 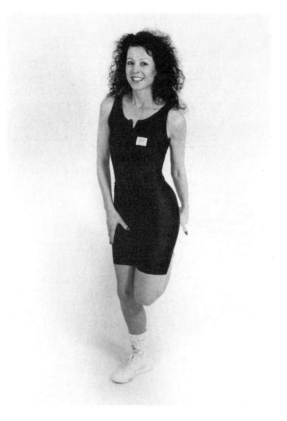

EXERCISE 58

You should end the aerobics section with a slow walk around the room, for between three to five minutes. Follow this with a couple of short stretches – just to ease the legs and the upper body – holding each one for about eight seconds (and no more). For example, you might want to stretch the front of the thigh, the calf muscle, the back of your upper leg, the shoulders, the upper back and the chest. This will safely return your heart and breathing rates to their natural levels.

Well done, you have now finished the aerobic section of your work-out. Now sip some water.

2 Using Weights

PREVENTION OF INJURY WHEN PERFORMING STRENGTH TRAINING

Points to Remember

1. Start with light loads and then gradually progress to larger loads (in the illustrations I am using 1lb/450g Spenco weights). For the first few weeks you should work without weights until you feel comfortable and confident in what you are doing.
2. Progress slowly – do not hurry.
3. Do not hold your breath.
4. Do not hyperventilate (breathe too quickly).
5. Do not use your back as a lever.
6. Avoid squatting too low.
7. Moves should be slow, controlled and with a definite rhythm.
8. Sip water often (to prevent dehydration).
9. Do not work out with weights when you have a fever, cold, hypertension, heart disease, recent surgery, hernia or back problems.
10. Always warm up and cool down.
11. Work all opposing muscle groups in order to prevent creating muscle imbalance.
12. Remember that muscles contract (pull) and relax (lengthen).
13. To see desired results, you should work out three times a week.
14. Do not swing your arms, especially when doing movements at shoulder height as this can cause injury.
15. Avoid hyperextension of your elbows: keep the elbow joint 'soft'.

POSTURE

When working with weights, you should always stand tall, your pelvis slightly tilted towards your navel (to get rid of any arch in your back), your stomach pulled in and your chest lifted – think tall. Your shoulders should be pressed back and down and you should breathe comfortably. Your legs should be hip-distance apart and your knees slightly bent. As you go through your exercises, periodically check your posture and maintain good body alignment.

How Often Should I Work Out?

As a rough guide, you should aim to build up to performing three sets of eight repetitions on each muscle group every other day – or at least three times a week. So far as the maximum amount you might do each day or each week is concerned – your own body will tell you in its own way. I predict that you will soon feel and respond to the 'challenge' of your muscles.

MYTHS ABOUT STRENGTH TRAINING

The following statements are, to varying degrees, widely held to be true by the public. In fact, all are false, and it is important to remember that they are incorrect – it can be dangerous to give them credence.

1. Women will gain a masculine, muscular physique.

2. Food supplements will speed up an increase in strength.
3. No pain, no gain.
4. A complete work-out requires two and a half hours.
5. Steroids are a safe and effective aid to strength training.

EXERCISE 59

Presses

Hold your weights shoulder height with your elbows bent and your palms facing down. Press your hands together but imagine that there is a beach-ball there and you are reaching around it. As you press together, feel the effort in the pectoral (chest) muscles and return to starting position.

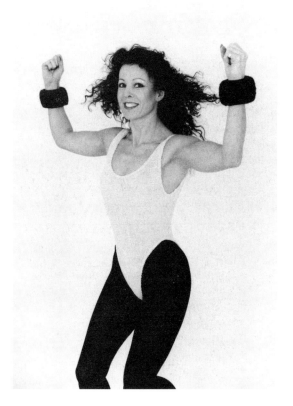

EXERCISE 60

Lift your elbows to shoulder height with the weights and your palms pointing towards the ceiling. Move your arms out to the side of your body and then return them to their starting position in front of your chest. Do two sets of eight.

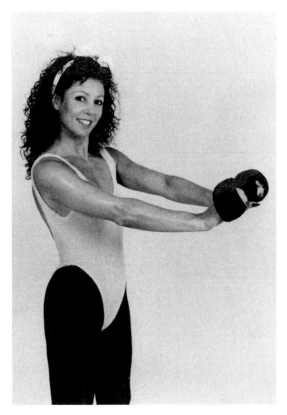 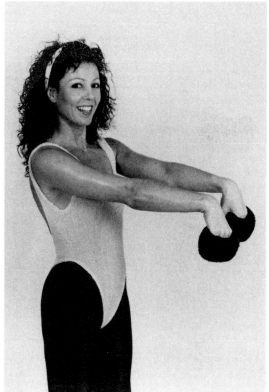

EXERCISE 61

Forearm Rotation

Stretch your arms straight out in front of your body, but without locking your elbows and holding the weights loosely. Slowly, for the count of four, roll your wrists to the right through a comfortable range of motion and again to the count of four to the left. Perform four repetitions in each direction.

EXERCISE 62

Forearm Press

Hold your arms as in the previous exercise and move your wrists slowly up and down, allowing the hand and weight to travel through a comfortable range of motion. Repeat this four times up and four down.

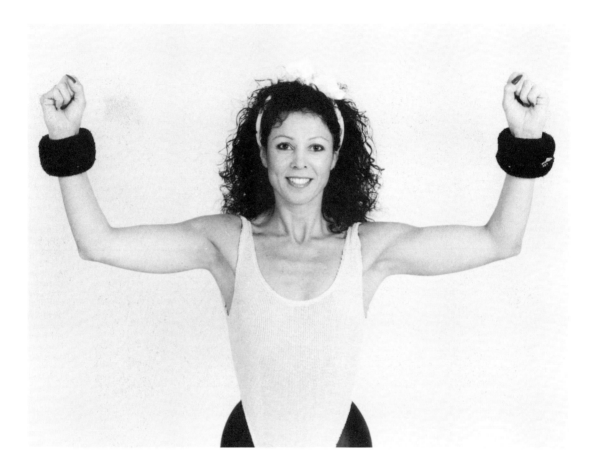

EXERCISE 63

Bicep Curls –
Front of the Arm

With your elbows at shoulder height and to the side of your body and with your palms facing your face, slowly curl your arms up towards you for a slow count of two and back to the starting position for a slow count of two. These movements should be done slowly and under control. Perform two sets of eight.

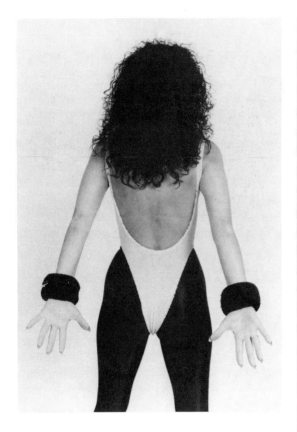

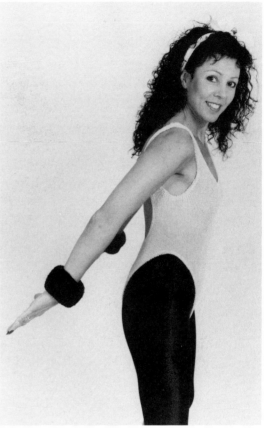

EXERCISE 64

Tricep Extension – Back of Upper Arm

Stand with a good posture; your back straight, your knees bent, your toes forward and your hips square and then bend both your arms so that your elbows point up and are behind your back. Without altering this position, slowly straighten your elbows without locking your elbow joints, press the weights back. Then slowly return to the starting position without bringing the elbows forward. Do two more sets of eight.

EXERCISE 65

Tricep Extension – Alternative

Extend your arms back so that your palms are facing the ceiling. Raise your palms up and back in a gentle, smooth, controlled motion. Feel the work in the back of the upper arm.

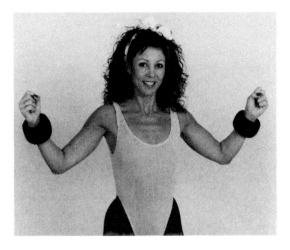

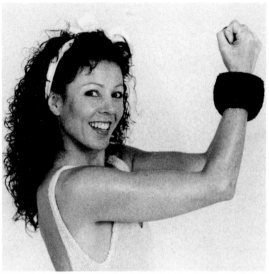

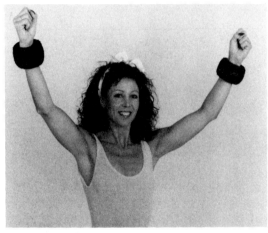

EXERCISE 66

Shoulder Press

This exercises the deltoid muscles in the middle of the back and the shoulders. Stand with a good posture; your knees slightly bent, your back in a straight line and your shoulders relaxed. Your arms are bent in front of your waist. Slowly and gently raise your arms behind your head and exhale. Do not lock your elbows when you have raised them and slowly lower them behind your head and inhale. Make sure you do not arch your back. Repeat four times.

EXERCISE 67

Pectorals Press

With your elbows at shoulder height and your palms facing each other, slowly bring your arms together for a slow count of two – then return to the starting position for two. Do two sets of eight.

A variation entails bringing the weights across your chest by crossing your elbows – so that the left weight is in front of your right shoulder and vice versa. Alternate having the left and right elbow nearest you and squeeze your chest muscles as you perform the exercise. Do sets of eight repetitions.

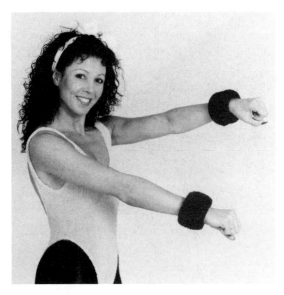
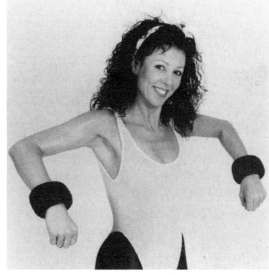

EXERCISE 68

Scissors (Vertical) Deltoids

Scissor the arms first up and then down for the count of two.

EXERCISE 69

Straight Arm Crosses

With your hands at shoulder level and both hands out in front of your body, palms facing each other, cross your arms, one over the other, alternating right over left, left over right. Do not create any momentum, but move your arms in a slow and controlled manner.

EXERCISE 70

Curls Triceps

Your elbows should be at shoulder height and your hand beneath your armpits. Slowly move your forearms out to the side of your body for a slow count of two, returning them for a further slow count of two under your armpits – making sure that when your arms extend fully to the side of the body, the elbows do not lock. Do two sets of eight repetitions.

71

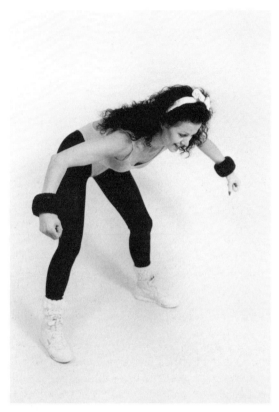 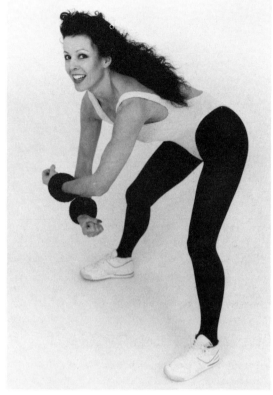

EXERCISE 71

Back Pulls (Lats and Trapezius Muscles)

Leaning forward to add to the work-load and with bent knees and a firm stomach, hold the weights out to the sides, your palms facing your body. Slowly lift up your elbows, pulling the weights to your chest and then slowly lower them again. Do two sets of eight repetitions.

EXERCISE 72

Back Flies (Lats and Trapezius Muscles)

Lean forward with a flat back, bent knees and your stomach pulled tight. Hold your arms at shoulder height, and your elbows slightly bent, then slowly lower your weights to the floor, your palms facing the body – then raise your arms up, pressing your shoulder-blades together.

When you finish your weights section, do some gentle shoulder rolls both forwards and backwards.

3 The Rubber-band Work-out

WHAT IS THE 'RUBBER-BAND' WORK-OUT?

For many years rubber-bands and/or surgical tubing have been used regularly by physiotherapists to strengthen injured muscles. While working in America in 1979 these rubber-bands attracted my attention and I started using them in my classes for a fun, proven, safe and effective work-out. They are a great way to firm, tone, strengthen and condition your body. They are also simple and portable and use the principle that when you overload a muscle it will strengthen.

Lie down on the floor on your back with one knee bent and one knee straight. Slowly lift your straight leg up and down; feel what it is like. Now, place the band around your ankles, lie in the same position and slowly lift your straight leg up and down; feel the difference.

Get to know your body and how to work out effectively. For the first couple of weeks you might want to work out without your bands until you become stronger. As you become stronger, start by using double bands (because you will be working with less tension – resistance – than with a single band). Indeed, every exercise shown in this book uses double bands – to make the work-out easier. When needed you can use the same exercise routine with the single band. To begin, try to work-out with bands three times a week for twenty minutes at a time.

SAFETY

Points to Remember

1. Always check your rubber-bands before every work-out for tears, holes and thinness from constant use.
2. Wear protective garments between the rubber bands and the skin – these should include socks or leg warmers and shoes when the bands are around your ankles. To protect your hands you can use training gloves or sweat-bands.
3. When exercising, never pull the band towards your face in case it should break. Always turn your head away.
4. Never be careless or relaxed about safety; you must control the band at all times, never sacrificing safety for speed. Use the correct posture and alignment throughout your exercise routine.
5. Breathe regularly, bringing a continuous flow of oxygen through steady inhalations and exhalations.
6. Drink water before, during and after your work-out to prevent dehydration.
7. If at any time you feel pain during the work-out – stop immediately. Pain is a sign that something is wrong and the movement should not be continued. If the pain persists after exercise you should consult your doctor.
8. Always keep your knees and elbows relaxed during movements; the locking of joints causes strains to the ligaments and tendons of the particular joint. Your shoulders should be relaxed at all times, especially with

upper-body moves (hunched shoulders create tension and cause an improper execution of moves).

9. Do not eat for at least two hours before exercise.

10. Control muscle contraction by maintaining a firm tension throughout your moves and with a full range of motion.

11. For the best results, in every exercise you should make sure the right and left sides of your body receive equal work.

12. Throughout your shape-up work at your own pace.

How to Hold the Bands

For most people the best way is to hold the band with clenched fists. Place the band across the palm with your fingers closed over it or, alternatively, you might prefer to hold the band with just a couple of fingers. It is up to you; try it and see what is comfortable. You can also alter the degree of resistance by changing the position of your grip; for example, for less resistance, grip the double band below the knot and for greater resistance, grip the double band on the knot (or make it even shorter).

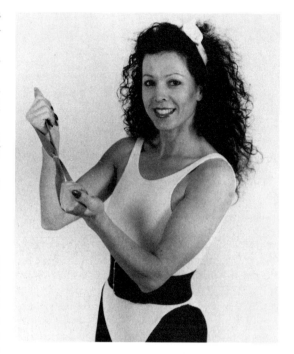

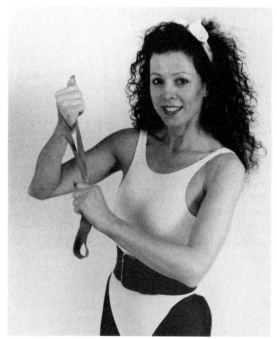

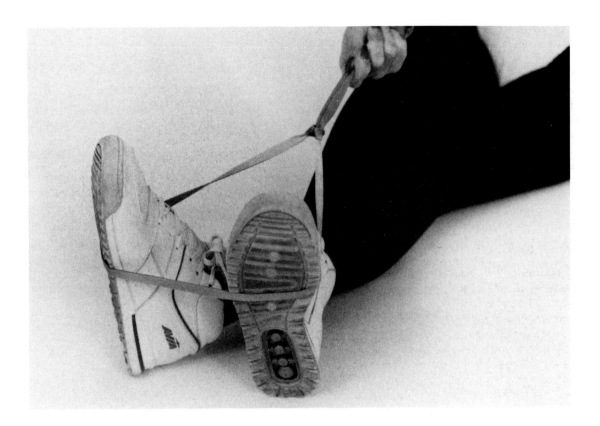

EXERCISE 73

Front of Lower Leg
(Tibialias Posterior)

Place the rubber-band under the soles of your feet. Hold on to the band and try to maintain tension, having crossed your legs at the ankles. Under control and keeping your toes pointed pull your feet apart and then return to the starting position. Do not let the band slacken.

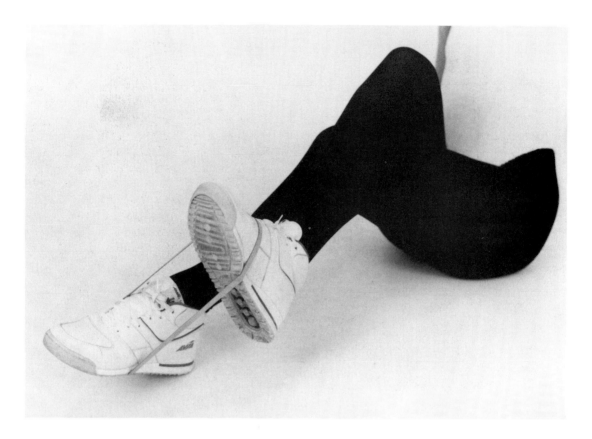

EXERCISE 74

Front of Lower Leg
(Tibialias Anterior)

Place the band over your feet as for the previous exercise. Then slowly pull your flexed foot towards your body and back again, keeping the band taut throughout.

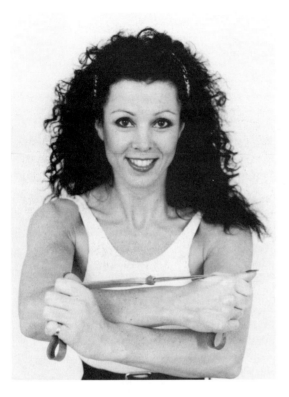

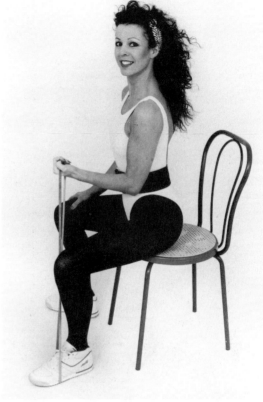

EXERCISE 75

Chest (Pectorals and Upper Torso)

Hold the double band by crossing your forearms as shown, then lift your arms to shoulder level and, under control, stretch the band so that your hands are further away from each other. Do two sets of eight and then cross your arms the other way and repeat.

EXERCISE 76

Front of Arm

Place one end of the double band under your right foot, and hold the other end in your right hand – across the palm and between the thumb and forefinger. Keeping your elbow into your waist and being careful not to let your hand turn downwards (which will put considerable amount of strain on your wrist) slowly curl your forearm up towards your shoulder. Do not lock your elbow as you straighten your arm and do not loosen the tension of the band. Do two sets of eight on the right arm and the same on the left.

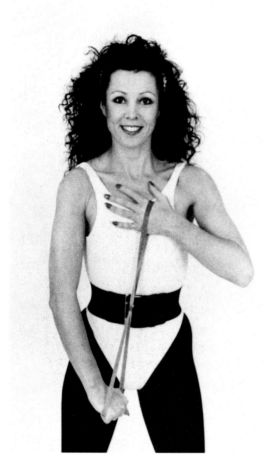

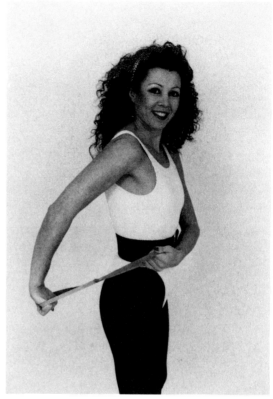

EXERCISE 78

Back of the Arm

This is an alternative means of firming the back of the arm. Adopt the basic standing position and then hold on to one end of the band, placing it at the right-hand side of your waist. Hold the other end of the band in your right hand with a fist grip, your palm facing backwards. Keeping your elbow pointed backwards and moving only your forearm, slowly and with control, push your right hand back as far as possible before slowly returning to starting position. Do two sets of eight and then change hand positions and repeat the exercises.

EXERCISE 77

Back of the Arm

Hold one end of the band in your left hand (as shown) against your chest and the other end in a fist grip. The left hand stays in its position whilst you press the right hand down towards the floor (without locking the elbow and without the elbow swinging out). Then release slowly, keeping the band taut. Repeat this between eight and sixteen times before changing hands.

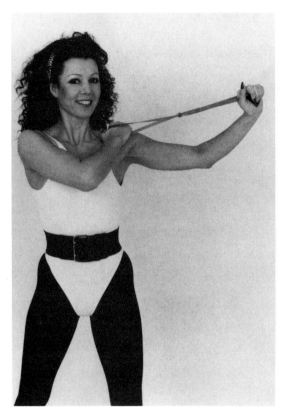 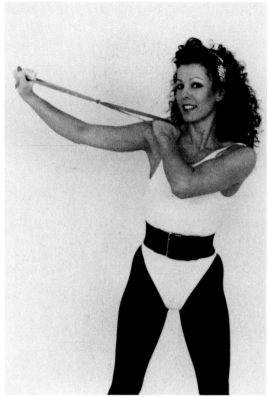

EXERCISE 79

Back of the
Arm Sideways Press

Adopt your correct standing position holding one end of the band in your right hand, which is on your right shoulder. At shoulder height, slowly push your left forearm out to the side and then return it without the band going slack. Switch hand positions and repeat the exercise with the left arm, in each case doing two sets of eight.

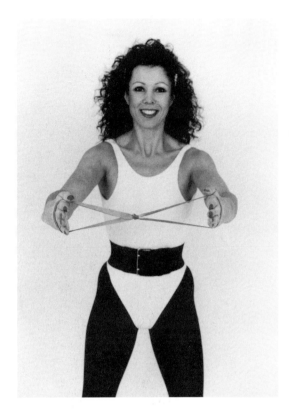

EXERCISE 81

Back and Shoulders

Keeping your weight evenly distributed, hold on to the bands with both hands and lift your elbows to your sides at chest height. Slowly, and under control, pull both hands apart while pressing your shoulder blades together. Release slowly, keeping complete control of the bands. Do two sets of eight.

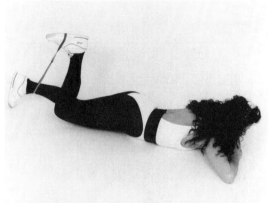

EXERCISE 80

Back and Shoulders

Extend your arms in front of your body at chest height and with your elbows slightly bent. Hold on to the bands with your palms facing towards each other and then apply outward pressure by pulling your hands apart. Do two sets of eight and then a further two sets of eight above your head.

EXERCISE 82

Back of Thigh

Adopt the basic prone position (head down, chin resting on your hands) and place one end of the band around your left ankle and the other end around the arch of your right (flexed) foot. Slowly and smoothly curl the right lower leg towards the buttocks and then slowly 'uncurl' it back to the starting position. Try to maintain pelvic and trunk stability throughout by contracting the abdominals – and so avoid any arching of your back. Do two sets of eight and then change the band position and exercise the other leg, again doing two sets of eight.

EXERCISE 83

Firming the Legs and the Bottom

The leg muscles are the most powerful of the body, especially those acting on the hip joint. This exercise is very effective when the bottom (gluteus maximus) is isometrically contracted. On one knee, with your elbows on the floor and the rubber-band around both ankles, raise the other leg and bend it at the knee. Flex your foot and slowly lift your leg up and down for two sets of eight counts. Maintain trunk and pelvic stability throughout the exercise and make sure you do not let your pelvis tilt forward as only about fifteen degrees of hyperextension is possible at the hip joint before the back arches.

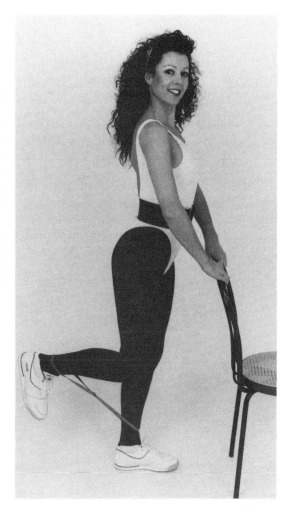

EXERCISE 84

Back of Thigh (Alternative position)

Using a chair stand tall with your stomach tucked in, straight back, bottom squeezed tight and rubber-band as shown. Flex your foot and then slowly curl your lower leg upwards before returning to the starting position. Keep controlled tension throughout the exercise.

81

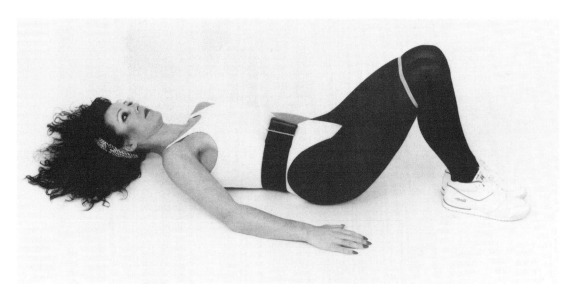

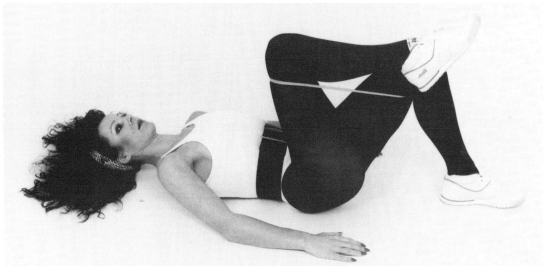

EXERCISE 85

Hip Flexor

Lie on your back and bend your knees as shown in the photograph. Push your spine into the floor and place your arms by your side. Place one band above both knees and slowly, under control, bring the right knee in towards your chest before returning to the starting position. Do eight to sixteen repetitions with each leg.

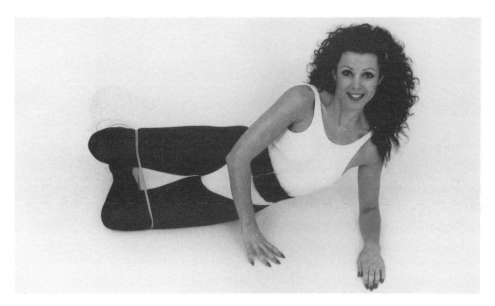

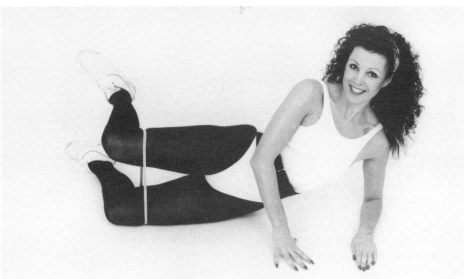

EXERCISE 86

Outer Thigh

Lie on one side of your body and place the double band around your thighs, keeping your hips and knees facing forwards. With both legs bent, slowly raise the top leg up towards the ceiling and then lower – but do not slacken the tension completely. Keep the repetitions smooth and continuous. Change sides and repeat the exercise, performing two sets of eight repetitions. Remember to keep the band above your knees if you have any knee problems.

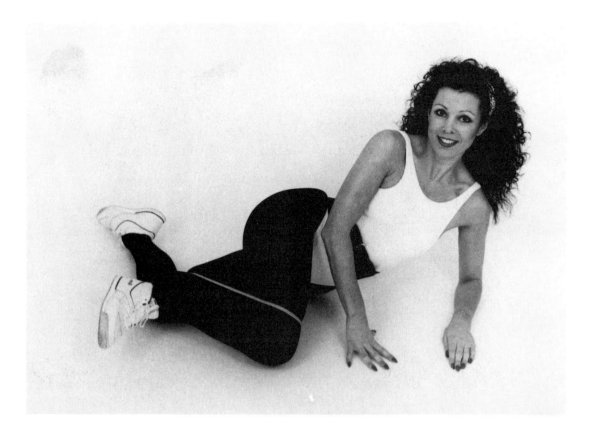

EXERCISE 87

Lie on one side as in the previous exercise with the double band around your thighs and your hip facing up towards the ceiling – you can raise your body on one elbow if you wish. Your supporting leg should be bent. Then slowly lift the top knee up and then forward to a spot on the floor in front of the abdomen to a slow count of four and return to the starting position. Do two sets of eight before switching your legs.

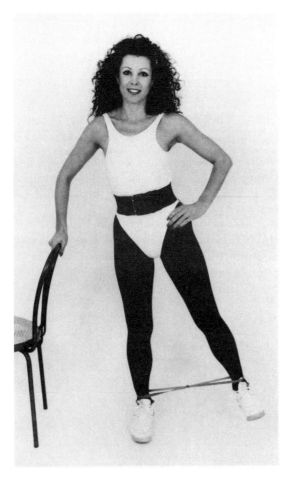

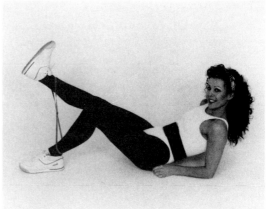

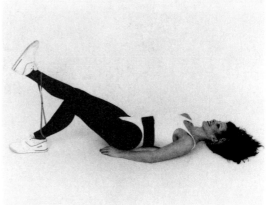

EXERCISE 88

Outer Thigh and Bottom (Alternative position)

Place the band around your ankles and hold on to a chair for balance while checking for the correct posture. Bend your knees slightly and tighten your stomach before slowly moving your leg to the side and then returning to the starting position without the band slackening off. Remember not to lean in towards the chair and to make sure you breathe regularly. Do sixteen repetitions on each leg.

EXERCISE 89

Front of Thigh and Hip

Lie back and either rest your weight on your elbows with your forearms on the floor or lie down completely. Place the band around both feet; one knee is bent with the foot flat on the floor. Extend the other leg – the working leg – and flex this foot, making sure you do not lock the knee joint. Keep your hips stable and pull your lower back to the floor, tucking in your pelvis and then slowly lift your leg up and down. Take two counts to lift up and two counts to go down, always keeping the band taut. Do two sets of eight repetitions.

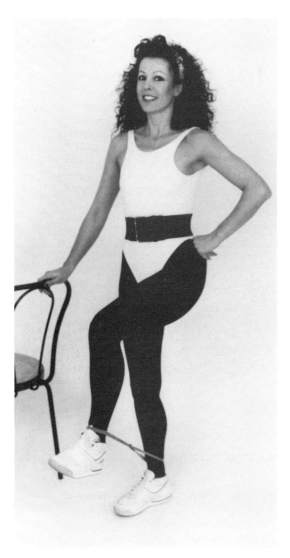

EXERCISE 90

Front of Thigh

Sit in a chair or hold on to the wall or back of a chair to help you keep your balance. Use a double band and place it around both ankles, then adopt a good posture, holding your stomach in and with your body in a straight line. The right (supporting) leg should be relaxed and your knee unlocked with both feet facing forward. Slowly lift the left knee up for five counts and hold this basic position throughout the exercise. Slowly, under control, extend the lower leg forward for five counts (without locking the knee joint) and then return to the starting position for five counts. Do two sets of eight repetitions before changing legs and repeating the exercise on the other leg. If you wish to make this exercise harder, you can raise your thigh a couple of inches.

4 Exercises for the Abdominal Muscles

A SELECTION OF SIMPLE ABDOMINAL EXERCISES (WITHOUT THE BANDS)

If you have not worked the abdominal muscles before, do not use the band as your body will provide more than enough resistance for these exercises. Abdominal work, to be effective, must be performed in such a way that it involves several different muscles:

1. the rectus abdominus;
2. the external obliques;
3. the internal obliques;
4. the transversus abdominus.

Levels of activity in abdominal work can be varied by where you position your arms – as this changes the centre of gravity of your upper body.

Selection of Moves

The following are basic moves which will be used in the exercises below:

1. reaching to knees with your hands;
2. supporting your head lightly with your hands and your elbows pressed back;
3. touching just by your ears with your fingertips, your elbows pressed back;
4. framing your face (not holding it) with your hands, with your elbows pressed back.

Note: when you have your hands near your head, do not clasp them round the back of your neck. This can cause injury by applying pressure to the top of your spine.

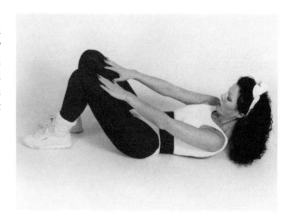

EXERCISE 91

The Rectus Abdominus (Centre)

These are slow abdominal exercises; the least difficult is the curl-up with your arms reaching forward to your knees. Lie on your back, pushing your spine down so that it is flat on the floor. Bend your knees and place both feet flat on the floor, hip-distance apart. Slowly lift your head and shoulders off the floor and reach towards your knees and then gently lower your head and shoulders; exhale on raising, inhale on lowering. Do two sets of eight and then rest.

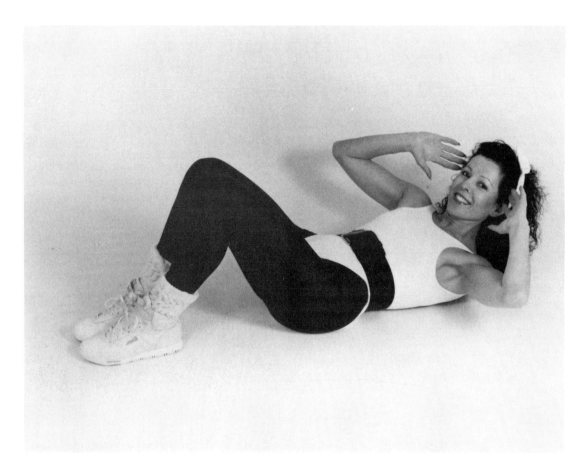

EXERCISE 92

This is a slightly more difficult exercise; stay in the position as before, frame your face with your hands and slowly lift your head and shoulders off the ground and back down again. Keep your back rounded throughout the exercise and try to keep your shoulder-blades off the floor. Do not relax the muscles in your abdomen; breathe regularly.

EXERCISE 93

This again is a more difficult abdominal exercise. Keeping in the same position as the previous exercise, cross your arms over your chest and, with your chin bent down, slowly curl up half-way – exhaling – keeping your head and shoulders off the floor before inhaling and lowering your head and shoulders. Do two sets of eight repetitions.

As you advance you can curl up to about ten degrees, hold for five quick counts, curl up for a further two degrees, hold for another five quick counts and slowly lower your head and shoulders to the floor before repeating. Always look for excellence in your technique and ensure you use controlled (and safe) movements.

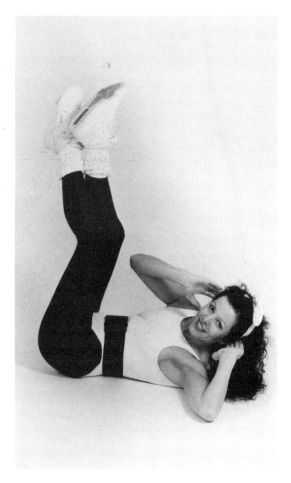

EXERCISE 94

The Obliques (Waist)

Lie down on your back as before, with your legs flat on the floor, then lift both legs into the air. Bend your knees slightly and make sure your feet are directly above your hips. Adding rotation to these abdominal curls will improve the oblique (waist) muscles.

When the exercises without the rubberband become easy, you can move on to incorporating it in your exercises.

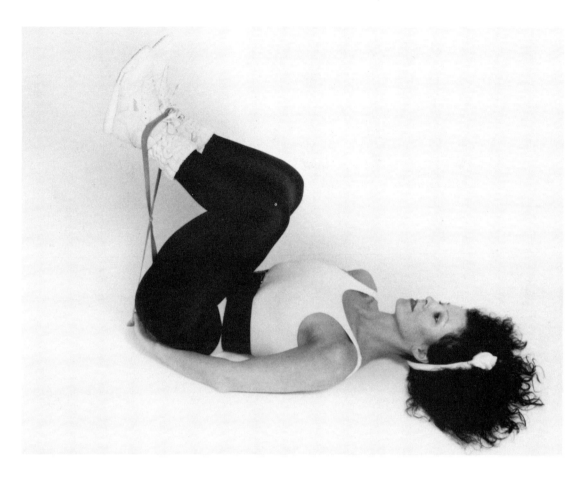

EXERCISE 95

Reverse Abdominal Curl-up

Lie on your back flat on the floor with your shoulders relaxed. Place one end of the double band around your ankles. Hold the other end of the band in your hands, which you should place under your buttocks as shown in the illustration. Slowly bend your knees to hip level and then on towards your chest; then move them back to hip level, but not past your hips. Do two sets of eight.

EXERCISE 96

Abdominal Obliques

Lie on your back with one end of the double band around your right ankle. Hold the other end in your right fist and bring your hands up under your head. Slowly, and under control, lift your upper body towards your left knee and then return to the starting position, keeping your shoulders off the floor. Do two sets of eight and change sides. Remember to keep your repetitions controlled and smooth.

SECTION 3
THE COOL-DOWN

1 Cool Down and Relax

It is important to emphasise the importance of flexibility and mobility of joints and the suppleness of muscles. The movements in this section should be smooth, slow and sustained – held for about thirty seconds to the point of tension, but not pain. Use slow, regular breathing to give a sense of complete relaxation and refreshment. Relaxation should aim to bring about a sensation of body and mind which is completely lacking in tension.

EXERCISE 97

Low Back Stretch

Lying on the floor, bring your knees up to your chest. Clasp your hands behind your thighs and gently pull them towards your chest, lifting your bottom off the floor. Tension should be felt in your hips and low back. Hold this position for about twenty or thirty seconds and breathe slowly and deeply. After the first fifteen seconds lift your head off the floor. Do not hold your breath – possible when you concentrate hard on something.

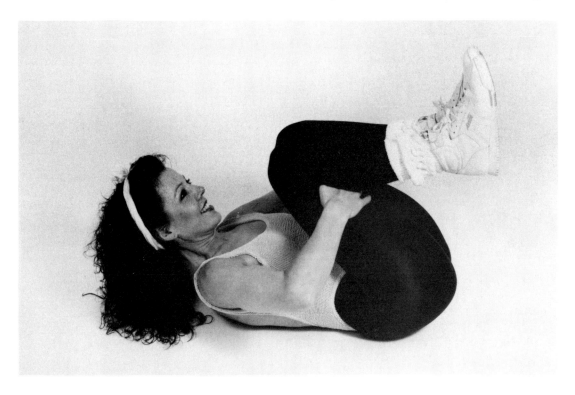

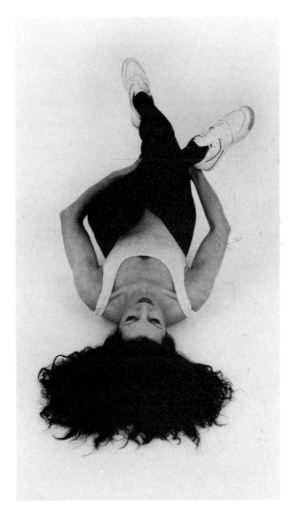

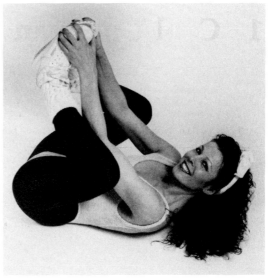

EXERCISE 99

Alternate Inner Thigh Stretch

Adopt the basic supine position, then bend your knees, placing the soles of your feet together as shown. Open your thighs and gently pull your feet in towards the centre of your body. You should feel the stretch in your inner thigh.

EXERCISE 98

Outer Thigh

Lying on your back, completely relaxed, bend your left leg and place your left foot over your right thigh just above the knee. Place your hands behind the back of your right leg and gently bring your legs towards your chest. Hold for twenty or thirty seconds and then change legs.

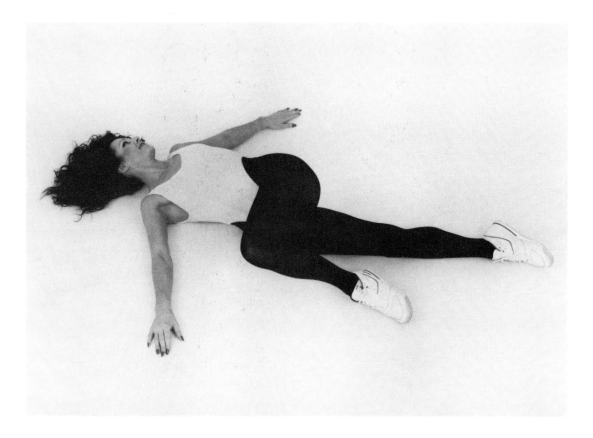

EXERCISE 100

Hips and Back

Lie on your back and relax your neck so that it is not arched. Move your arms out to the side of your body and then slowly take your left knee over your right leg (you might need to give it a gentle press down). Relax your extended leg and keep both shoulders flat on the floor. This stretch will be felt on the left side of your lower back and along the top of your buttocks. Hold for about thirty seconds and change sides.

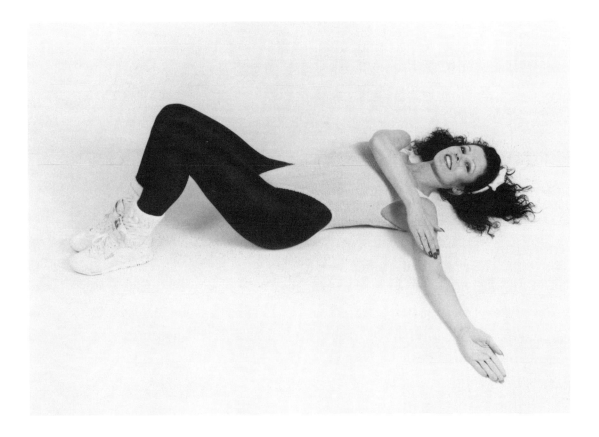

EXERCISE 101

Shoulder and Upper Back

Adopt the basic supine position, with your knees bent and your feet apart. Allow your knees to relax and lean one against the other, then push your spine down into the floor and extend one arm at shoulder-height to the side. Reach and stretch the other arm across the body, your shoulders staying on the floor. Hold for about thirty seconds before repeating on the other side.

EXERCISE 102

Bend both knees and keep your buttocks and shoulders on the floor. Then slowly arch your lower back and gently push it towards the floor; your pelvis should 'rock' up and down slowly. Breathe regularly.

EXERCISE 103

Lie on the floor as for the last few exercises, but then let your knees fall back on to the floor and use your arms to push yourself up into a sitting position. Now continue your stretches in this position.

Remember that stretching is not competitive and that each individual has a different ability. Never stretch too far, never hold your breath when stretching and never 'bounce' at the end of your stretches. In general, exhale as you stretch and breathe as normal when holding a particular position.

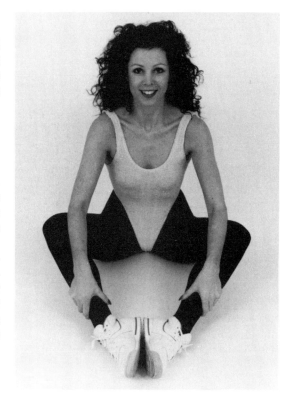

EXERCISE 104

Groin Stretch (Inner Thigh)

Sit on the floor and bring your feet together so that your soles touch. Place your elbows by the insides of your flexed knees, hold your ankles and lean forward, pressing down gently on them. Push your knees together and towards the floor slowly and under control. Hold for between ten and thirty seconds; gentle tension will be felt inside your upper legs. If you feel the stretch is too difficult for you, take your feet further out in front of you and again bend forward from the hips until you feel a mild stretch in the groin. Throughout this exercise, you should aim to keep a straight back.

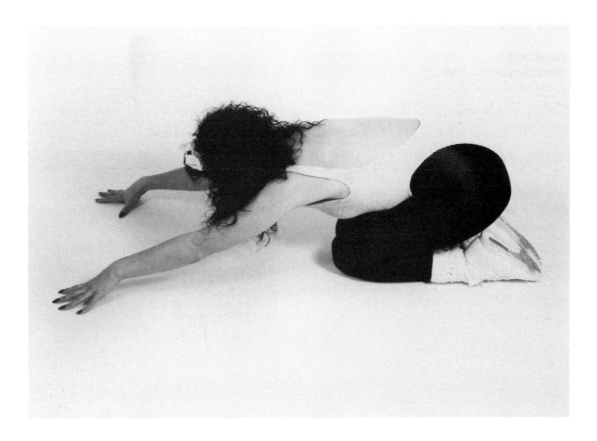

EXERCISE 105

Cat Stretch

Sit on your knees and lean forward with your arms outstretched. Stretch your back forward until a position of slight tension is reached and hold this for thirty seconds before slowly returning to the starting position.

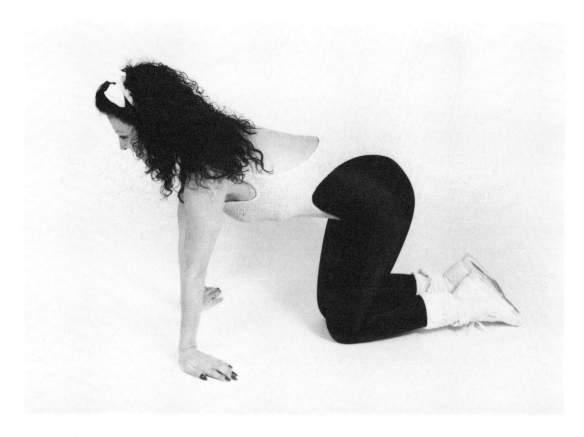

EXERCISE 106

Wrist and Forearm Stretch

Take up the position on all fours, as shown. Keep your palms flat on the floor with your thumbs slightly turned out. Slowly move your body-weight back until slight tension is felt in the wrists and forearms. Hold for about thirty seconds.

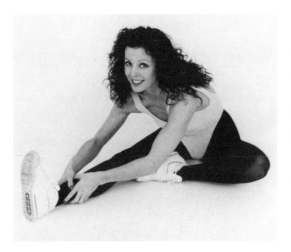

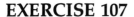

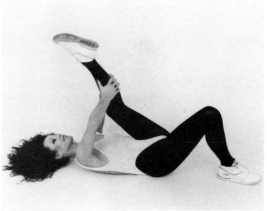

EXERCISE 107

Back of the Leg (Hamstring) Stretch

In a sitting position with one leg straight and one leg bent, rest the sole of your foot against your straight leg. Your relaxed knee and toe should both face the ceiling. Slowly bend from your hips, leaning forward and taking your abdomen towards your thigh. Tension will be felt along the back of your thigh. Make sure your knee joint is not locked – indeed it is quite acceptable to keep your knee slightly bent.

EXERCISE 108

An Alternative Hamstring Stretch

This is suitable for people with less flexibility in the back of the leg and lower back. Push down your spine on to the floor so that there is no gap between your back and the floor, with one leg bent and the other straight. Grab the straight leg below or above the knee and gently pull the leg towards your chest, slowly and under control. Hold for thirty seconds when there is tension but no pain in your hamstring, then change legs. If you feel this stretch is too difficult, hold your bent knee near your chest and do not move it. Then slowly extend the lower leg. You should feel the tension in the back of your upper leg.

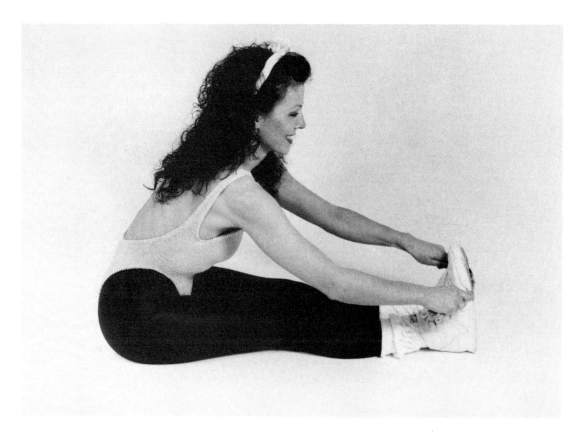

EXERCISE 109

Alternative Hamstring Stretch (Seated)

Sit on the floor with your legs fully stretched out in front of you and place the band around your feet. Slowly lean forward from your hips, keeping your back and neck in a straight line; you will feel a stretch in the back of your legs. Again, stretch and hold for about thirty seconds.

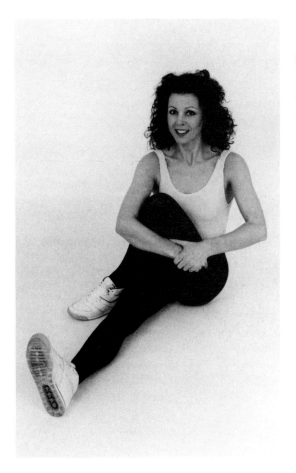

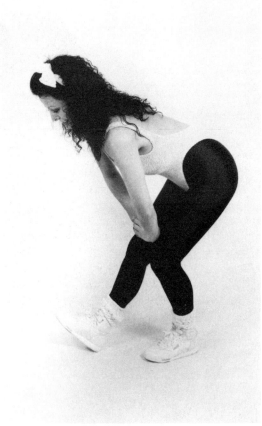

EXERCISE 110

Alternative Hip Stretch

Sit on the floor with your back straight and extend your right leg, toes pointing to the ceiling, while the left leg crosses over your right leg. Place your left foot on the floor next to your right leg between the knee and the hip and wrap your right arm around the lower left leg and gently pull your left knee towards the opposite shoulder. Slight tension will be felt in the hip and buttock of the bent leg. Hold for thirty seconds and then change legs.

EXERCISE 111

Alternative Hamstring Stretch

Stand with your feet staggered, shoulder-distance apart and place your hands on your thighs for support. Bend your back knee and raise the toes of your front foot until you feel a stretch in the rear of the thigh. To increase the stretch, place more body-weight on the back heel. Hold the stretch for about thirty seconds before returning to the starting position and repeating with the other leg.

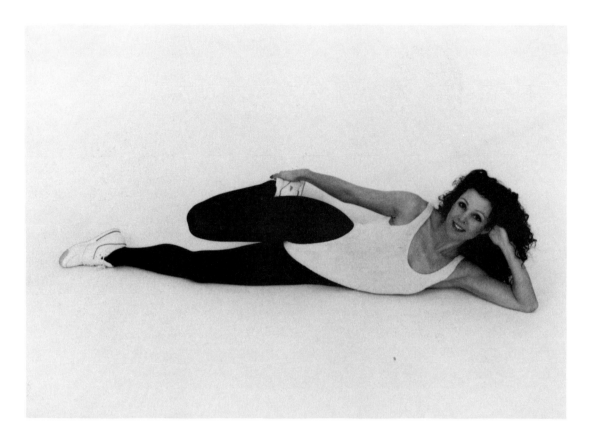

EXERCISE 112

The Thigh

Lie on your side, propping yourself up on one elbow, but not letting your pelvis tip forward. Bring the heel of your top leg up towards your buttocks and feel the stretch in the front of the thigh. More of a stretch can be added by pushing your foot into the hand. Hold for thirty seconds, change legs and repeat.

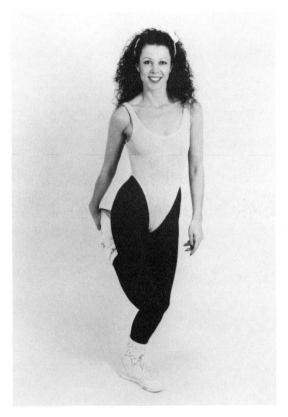

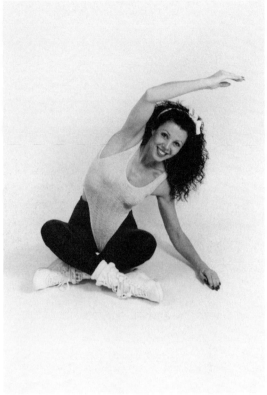

EXERCISE 113

Alternative Quad Stretch

Stand tall with a good posture – your shoulders relaxed, knees slightly bent, stomach tucked in and breathing comfortably. Slowly lift one foot up towards your bottom (hold your foot loosely and ease it gently towards you). The stretch should be felt in the front part of your upper leg and you should feel no pressure at the knee. Hold for thirty seconds and then change legs.

EXERCISE 114

Torso Lift

Sit on the floor with your ankles crossed in front of you. Then place one hand on the floor close to your hips, making sure that your elbow is slightly bent, and not locked. Extend your other arm above your head in line with your shoulder. Breathing comfortably, lift the upper body up and slowly lean forwards and across on to your bent elbow. Hold for twenty or thirty seconds before changing sides.

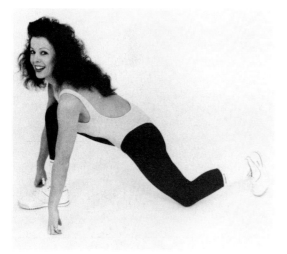 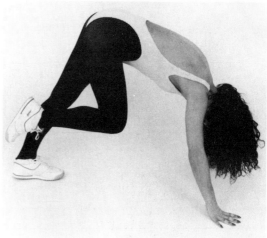

EXERCISE 115

Hip Flexors and Thighs

Crouch on the floor on all fours and position your front leg as in the illustration, so that your knee is bent at ninety degrees and it is directly above your ankle. Keep your stomach tight and make your back as long as possible. Bend your back leg slowly until tension is felt in your upper thigh and push your hips forward, making sure the weight is not on your knee-cap. Hold for a count of twenty or thirty seconds and then change legs.

EXERCISE 116

Calf Stretch

Bend down and put both your hands on the floor in an A-frame position. Lift your right leg off the floor – or just rest it in front of the ankle of your left foot. Immediately you will feel your calf muscle in your straight leg being stretched. Keep your heel down, your toes pointed straight ahead and relax your knee. If the stretch is too much for you (remember you should feel tension and not pain) narrow the A-frame by moving your hands closer to your feet and making the stretch comfortable. Hold for thirty seconds and then change legs.

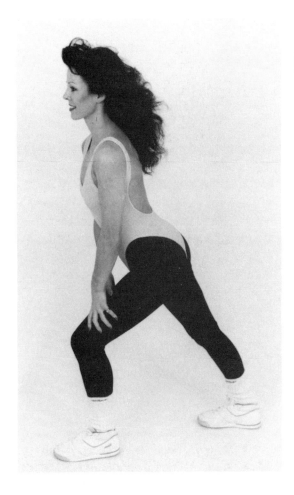

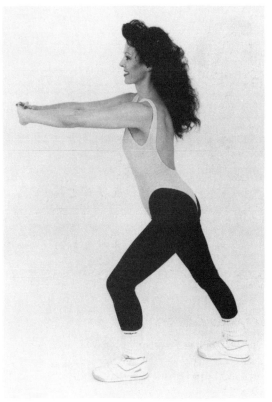

your toes, both heels pressed down towards the floor. Hold the stretch, which is felt along the calf, until a feeling of tightness changes to a feeling of released tension. Again, you should feel no pain. Your hands can either be placed on your thigh or extended in front of your chest. Hold for about thirty seconds and change legs.

EXERCISE 117

Calf Stretch
(Alternative position)

Stand with your torso leaning forward and your stomach held in, keeping your head, upper body, chest and stomach in line as much as possible. Bend the front knee and feel the weight of your body over your front leg – your other leg is extended back with a 'relaxed' knee. Keep your toes pointing straight ahead and your heels directly behind

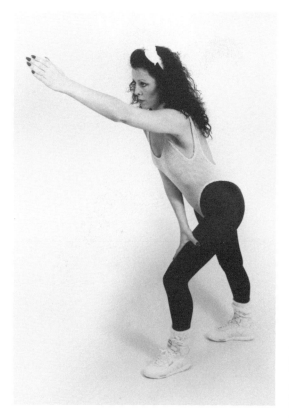

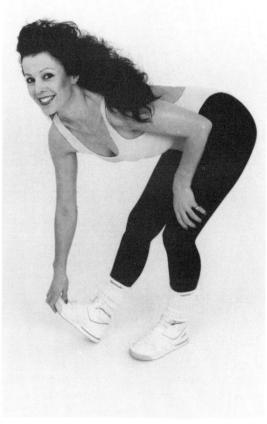

EXERCISE 118

Runner Stretch

Stand with your feet in a lunge position, both feet facing forward. Your hips should be square, buttocks tucked, stomach tight – but do not arch your back. Bend your front knee until the lower leg is perpendicular to the floor (keeping the heel of your back foot on the floor) and then lift the opposite arm as if to lengthen your spine. Hold the stretch for twenty to thirty seconds and then return to the starting position and repeat with your other leg.

EXERCISE 119

Back of Lower Leg

Firm your stomach and bend your knees, then slowly bend forward from the hip, resting your toes in your hand and raising them towards your shin. A slight stretch will be felt in the lower calf. Hold for twenty or thirty seconds and change legs.

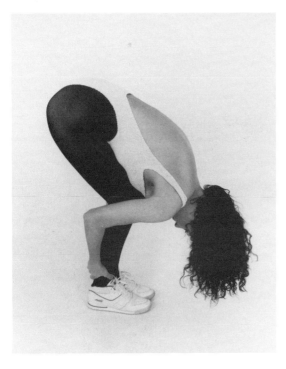

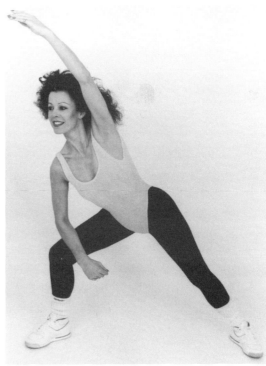

EXERCISE 120

Back of the Leg Stretch

Stand tall, with your stomach tucked in and knees slightly bent (to protect your back). Slowly curve your head down, bending your back vertebra by vertebra, and flexing your knees until your hands reach your ankles. Keep your rib-cage close to your thighs and slowly straighten your left leg, taking care not to lock the knee. Hold this position for ten counts and release. Change legs and straighten your right leg. After you have stretched both legs place your hands on the floor, weight on hands, and bend your knees as far as you can comfortably manage. Feel the stretch along the back of your legs. Straighten your knees gently, round your back, 'suck in' your stomach and uncurl to an upright position. If your hands cannot quite reach the floor, try using a step or perhaps two telephone books.

EXERCISE 121

Inner Thigh

Stand with your legs apart and put your weight on to your right thigh, lifting your left arm over your head. Your flexed knee should be directly above your ankle and the toes of your straight leg pointing forward – as shown in the illustration. When performing this exercise, there are some other points that you should bear in mind. Always remember to support your body, while keeping your buttocks and abdominal muscles tight. Remember also that when leaning to the side and stretching your spine you should not lean either forwards or backwards. You should aim to push your hips forward and create a long, straight line with your body, from toes to fingers. Hold this position for about thirty seconds before slowly returning to the starting position and repeating on the other side.

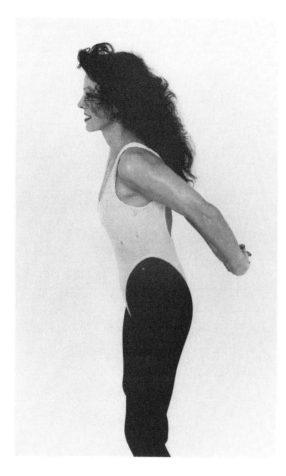

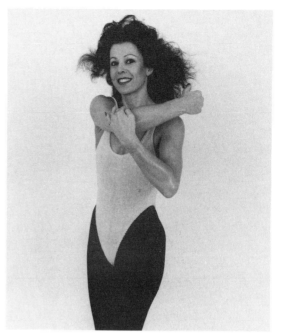

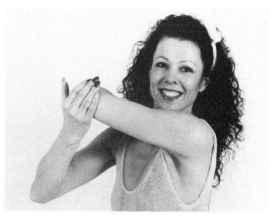

EXERCISE 122

Chest Stretch

Stand upright with your knees bent and then move your hands behind your back and interlock your fingers. Lift your arms up until slight discomfort is felt in the shoulder, chest and upper arms. Hold this for about thirty seconds and then return to the starting position.

EXERCISE 123

Alternative Shoulder Stretches

Hold your right arm just above the elbow with your left hand and gently pull the elbow towards your left shoulder. Do not hold your breath but breathe regularly. Hold this for thirty seconds and change sides.

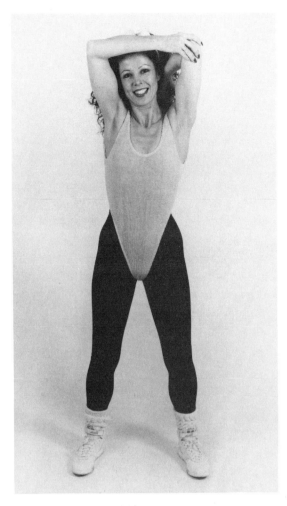

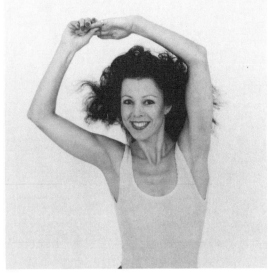

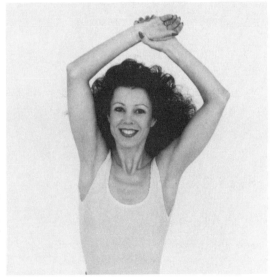

EXERCISE 124

Tricep Stretch

Tricep stretches exercise the back of the upper arm and the front and middle of the shoulders. Adopt the correct stance (your feet shoulder-width apart, knees soft, buttocks firm). Place one hand on the same shoulder, elbow pointing forward, and your other hand under the elbow. Lift your arm overhead, so pulling your shoulders back. Hold for about twenty to thirty seconds before changing arms and repeating.

EXERCISE 125

Shoulders and Arms

Raise your arms over your head and then take your left hand in your right and gently pull it to the side, feeling a stretch under the arm and shoulder. Hold for thirty seconds before changing sides.

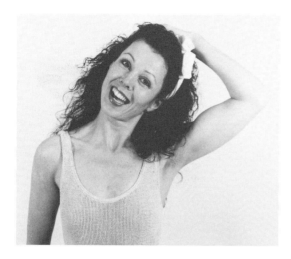

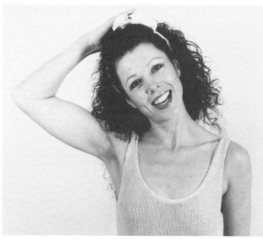

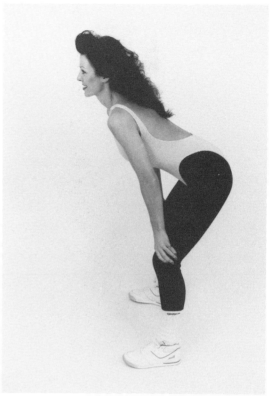

EXERCISE 127

Lower Back Stretch

Stand with your feet hip-distance apart, lean forward and place your hands on the thigh, just above your knees. Take a deep breath and slowly round your back as much as possible – with your stomach pulled in and your pelvis 'tilted under'. Exhale and slowly resume a flat-back position. Be careful not to arch your spine too much as you straighten your back.

EXERCISE 126

Neck Stretch

Stand in an upright position with your stomach tight, shoulders relaxed and chin tucked in. Bend your knees slightly and then tilt your head to the side, moving your ear to your shoulder, and gently resting one hand on the side of your head. Now gently pull your head to create a stretch down the side of your neck and shoulder. Hold for thirty seconds and then return your head to an upright position and change sides.

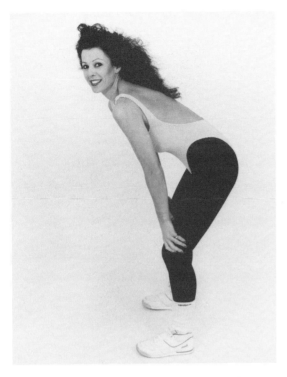

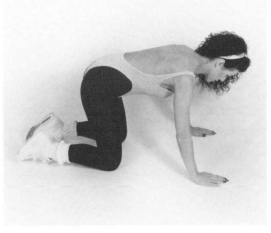

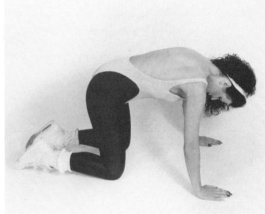

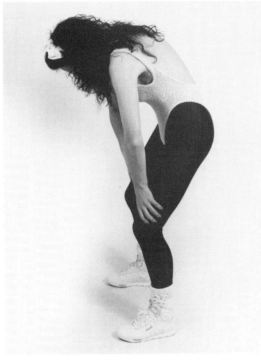

EXERCISE 128

Alternative Back Stretch

Kneel on all fours with your knees directly below your hips. Place your hands below your shoulders and keep your elbow joints soft, then slowly round your back and 'suck in' your stomach. Inhale and hold this position before exhaling and returning to a flat-back position.

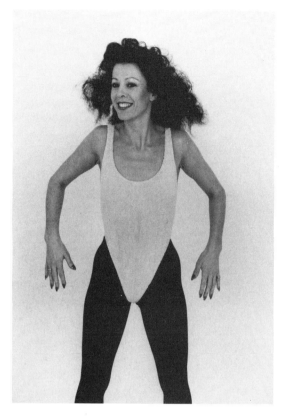
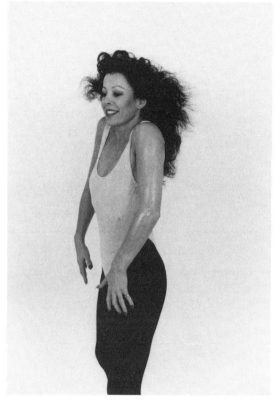

EXERCISE 129

Shoulder Shrugs

Begin by standing with a good posture, your arms loose to your side. Make sure your head is 'aligned' correctly by keeping your ears directly over your shoulders and your chin and jaw relaxed. Then bring your shoulders up, lifting your shoulder-blades and slowly lower them again. Take four counts for your lift and four to lower them.

. . . and to finish off your work-out, you should do some step-touches, simple walks, heel presses – indeed any movement to get your body going slightly – a revitaliser. Well done, you have finished your work-out!

112